JOURNAL
from an
OBSCURE
PLACE

JOURNAL
from an
OBSCURE
PLACE

JUDITH MILES

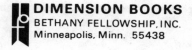

DIMENSION BOOKS
BETHANY FELLOWSHIP, INC.
Minneapolis, Minn. 55438

Journal from an Obscure Place
by Judith Miles

ISBN 0-87123-273-1

DIMENSION BOOKS
Published by Bethany Fellowship, Inc.
6820 Auto Club Road, Minneapolis, Minnesota 55438

Printed in the United States of America

Dedication

To Harold Keables, my high school English teacher.

Judith M. Miles

Mrs. Miles describes herself, with characteristic modesty, as a woman who "has astoundingly received grace and mercy from the Lord despite her resurgent pride of intellect and hardness of heart."

But there is much more to her personal story than this self-effacing summary:

She was born in Michigan, lived through her teens and twenties in Colorado, and spent several years in upstate New York.

She is married (happily) and the mother of three teenage children.

Mrs. Miles took her B.A. (cum laude) in English Literature from the University of Colorado, was elected to Phi Beta Kappa, and has a master's degree from the same institution. She has also done doctoral study in English Literature at the University of Denver.

A member of the Lutheran Church-Missouri Synod, she is usually involved in two or three church-related activities at any given time and in addition has been a foster parent to teenagers.

Judith Miles is the author of two other books: *Mind Games and Hobby Horses* and *The Feminine Principle*.

Contents

"In the Beginning . . . "

To my dear, unknown child with love. I am writing this journal of your first days for you, because you will have no way of knowing about them since your memory of these days will evaporate like the dew in childhood's sunshine. But you may wonder about your beginnings when you are older, for I know you are a perceptive and reflective child. Forgive me if I've said too much for you—or too little. Maybe you knew all of this in your spirit; maybe none. Some of your early weeks I remember only vaguely, for I was a different person then. Love your *real* mother and father for me, won't you? I mean the man and woman who have given a large portion of their lives over to caring for you. I will resist the impulse to give you all kinds of further advice from

Your Natural Mother

The First Week—The Seed

I begin my life on a November night not far, in cosmic perspective, from the fortieth parallel on the earth. The earthly desire that begot me was unholy, but the Heavenly Desirer who planned me is the Holy One. He allowed, for His own reasons, the miracle of me to be conceived in sin. From the very first I am a creature allowed by pure grace—an object of His mercy and love in a bad situation. You might say He made good use of a bad scene and produced life from a phase of death.

I sense that my parents love, but not enough. I don't know what human love is like yet, but I hope it is an emanation of the powerful, creative Love that is calling me together. I am bathed in the essence of Love now. Love was the compelling force that brought together the chosen sperm with the chosen egg to ignite *me* in a moment of time, in a measure of space. Love transcended the immediate, unhappy circumstances to make a good result—me—even though, I hear, Love prefers to create within the protected sanctity of the marriage bed, because Love desires to spare parents from the intense soulish pain that comes with any other arrangement. But one of Love's names, I heard whispered abroad, is Redeemer. So Love redeemed an awkward sadness in a borrowed bed, this cold November night, by bestowing precious, explosive *life* on me.

I am the size of a pinprick—a tiny egg that has received half its being from my earthly father's urgent life. Yet in my microscopic self I hold the full potential of my unique personhood; nothing more need be added but nourishment. I am the seed. But I am perishable seed, and I am vulnerable to the will of my earthly parents. Though I have every human possibility within me, I am frail and totally dependent on the body and soul of the woman who holds me.

I am, even now, from a timeless perspective, that which I will become. In my seed is the seed of Abraham, of a learned Greek, of a sea captain, of a devout mother of sixteen children, of a concert oboist, of a gymnast, of a farmer, of a lawyer, of a seamstress, of an errant military man, of a God-fearing pioneer, of an Indian maid. What shall I be like? Whose heart shall I delight?

Every complex alive thing, great and small, must begin as I did from a fertilized seed, a kernel of potent life. Whom can I thank for beginning *me* this way? I did not exist before. Now I do. What greater contrast could there ever be? Life or non-life says it all. I thank you, Love. May I call you Love until I learn your proper name? I thank you very much, Love.

My seed is completely programmed for my orderly development through my individualized combinations of chemical substances called genes. My myriad genes are contained in twenty-three pairs of chromosomes, one of each matched pair contributed by Mother and one by my Father. Since I am normal and Mother is physically able to carry me, I will grow without fail to be a perfect filled-out person on schedule, if no external evil interferes. My full person-potential is here in this little ball of cells—my seed has divided several times already. Earlier this week an angelic census taker has duly recorded my position, parentage, and propensities. I am *alive* and living in some obscure place!

The Second Week—The Tee Shirt

Someone called me "Blastocyst." I surely hope that is not my permanent name! The ball of cells that holds my future is forming a hollowed-out area. My cells are beginning to take differing shapes that will make my different parts. I am developing an inner cell mass, a thickening in one part of my physical self. At one end of the thicker part is my primitive streak. But now this primitive streak in me shows a cell difference; I am growing a neural plate, soon to be a neural groove. My neural groove will grow into my brain; I have a tiny rod of tissue that will be my spinal cord. The brain part of me is growing faster than the other parts now. The head must come first, and the body follows. I think this is a principle of growth. Now I am a microscopic picture of a pattern; the Head leads the Body.

I have a question I need to ask. I wonder if I am the very center of the universe. The reason I ask is that although I am so tiny—merely a speck— everything around me in this obscure place is changing drastically in order to nurture and preserve me. It is as though I were the most important speck ever created. Mother's hormones have taken on a new direction and purpose, and all of her body is concentrated on caring for me. And she doesn't even know that I am here. I am, in physical terms, just a blob so far.

Mother is wearing a tee shirt that has the words "My Body Belongs to Me" written on it in blue letters. I don't understand that. Wasn't she formed within her mother the same way I was? Didn't Love sunburst her into sudden, glorious life too? Could she make herself? Doesn't the one who creates something own it forever? Perhaps she believes that her mother and father own her, though they were merely agents in the making of her. Perhaps she's arguing against their ownership with that slogan. If she feels that her mother and father own her, then she would also feel that she owns me (when she discovers me) and could do what she wanted to with me. But I won't worry. Mother is very independent. I know that she doesn't feel that her parents own her!

I gather that Mother has a beautiful body to live in and it seems to function well. Love has given her breath for nineteen sun-years—that's about a hundred-forty-million person breaths. Each one was a free gift to her. I believe Love has fed her body every day of those years, sometimes with breast milk, sometimes with peanut butter sandwiches, sometimes with fast food and onion rings. I know that Love has healed her frequently—I'm becoming acquainted with her antibodies at a discreet distance. And her guardian angel should have retired long ago from exhaustion and nervous prostration if he were not indefatigable and unflappable.

From what I can observe, in many ways Mother's body operates independently from her conscious will. She cannot grow even another inch (upward) by thinking about it. She cannot control sickness or deterioration beyond her ability to practice good health measures. Most of her vital bodily functions are taken care of for her by her intricately designed, marvelously engineered body. She does not plan each heartbeat or metabolic conversion. In fact, all goes on very well when she is asleep. Right now her body is mobilizing for a totally unselfish purpose, not for its own preservation, but for me.

No, I don't believe that Mother's body belongs to

her, despite the blatant tee shirt. From my limited experience, it appears to me that her body must belong to Love who desired her into being and who sustains her life each moment. Love is the only One I would want to own me. In fact, I am so dazzled by Love's gift to me of erupting, glowing life that if I did think I owned myself I would throw myself at Love's feet in gratitude and give myself back to Love. Doesn't Mother know Love anymore? I guess I must wait to understand. Meanwhile, I will snuggle in under the tee shirt and allow my pre-programmed growth to proceed. I think this must be the coziest place in the vast, personal universe.

The Third Week—
The Writing Finger

I have a heart that beats! My heart pumps through a circulatory system, even though the total of me is one-tenth of an ounce. I am growing umbilical vessels that will allow Mother's body to nourish me. Love created my heart to function first because without the heart no other part of me can function. The rest of me can grow when my heart provides movement or motive power for my vital blood to circulate. Love uses the same word—heart—as a picture word when He tells me about that deep part of me where my spirit and soul meet, the spring of my personhood and my spiritual motive center. That is where Love is writing His order even now. Love is taking forty days to complete the writing into the very structure of my heart of flesh. After forty days of life the temporary vitelline circulatory system with my rudimentary heart will have developed into the placental circulatory system with my lifetime complex heart.

I have discovered that Mother is not living in her permanent home. She is attending a college that is supposed to prepare her for self-supporting Life in the World. She lives in a dormitory with a lot of other girls, all of whom seem to be older than seventeen sun-years. She goes to classes, eats three nutritious meals every day (when she gets up for breakfast), and spends most of her time talking in an animated way with other people. She hasn't spoken to me yet.

Look how Love is writing on my unscarred physical heart! My heart will be in two parts, like two stone tablets, side by side. My heart will have ten major openings through which my lifeblood will flow, hopefully unrestricted all my days. The right side of my heart will be like a tablet that faces Love, open and waiting to receive life. The left side will be like a tablet open for other people to read me. The right half will have four large openings—two entry gates, one valve between the upper and lower chambers, and one exit to the passageway to the lungs. The left side of my heart will have six major openings— four entryways from my air-touching lungs, one valve between chambers, and one floodgate to the vast aorta. I feel you writing now, Love. I love your order. Teach me. Write on and on. And after my forty days of being written on, quicken me to understand. When you have finished writing your law on my physical heart, O my Creator, my spiritual heart may understand too.

The right side of my heart will receive the blood from every part of my body through the two vein openings into the top part, the auricle. The third opening Love is making in the right part of my heart is the tricuspid valve between the auricle on top and the ventricle below. The valve opening is growing into three parts which form one ring at their base. It is like a name that has three parts, yet is one.

The fourth opening on the right tablet of my heart is for the pulmonary artery. The blood leaves my right ventricle through this opening and is propelled by my heartbeat to a time of rest and refreshment—a revitalization in the lungs where oxygen, the breath of life, will be absorbed by my blood (after I can breathe). This fourth opening to the area of my blood's rest and renewal is teaching me about a rest period for all that lives. My blood is in the reviving pulmonary cycle for one-seventh of the time. Thank you, Love, for making a time of rest and refreshment. Mother seems to know about the six-to-one-activity-to-rest principle because she sleeps real late every seventh day.

Of the six major openings in the left tablet of my heart, four are the pulmonary veins which will carry the oxygenated blood from my lungs to the left auricle of my heart; until I am born they return the blood that has been sent to nourish my growing lungs. The ninth opening in my heart is another one-way valve, the bicuspid valve between my left auricle and my left ventricle. The tenth major opening is for the aorta, the artery that will carry renewed blood out to nourish my many parts. This is the mainspring of my heart's ministry to the rest of the body. This opening is large to allow my life supply to surge outwards. I am impressed that this opening must never become constricted with junk or I might die. My heart can never supply nourishment and allow life to flow if it grasps and desires for itself.

Since I am dependent on Mother for my oxygen supply while I live in here, most of my blood will bypass openings five through ten until the day I am born into my outer life in the world with other people. You, my Holy Creator, are the only one I know now. Until I am born You have made a duct between my pulmonary artery and my aorta so that most of my blood is not concerned with openings five through ten. That duct will close with clotted blood at my birth and will become a fibrous cord. And, Love, You have made a way of *direct communication* between the two tablets of my heart, the Love-ward tablet and the people-ward tablet; the opening is called the *foramen ovale*. This opening will close shortly after my birth, never to reopen. Oh, no. Love, does this mean that after I am born my life with You no longer will be directly connected with my perceptions of the outside world and my life there with other people? Will I become like Mother who talks to everyone else but You? Oh, Love, Love, keep my heart always open to You. *I* love *You!*

You are writing your order on my heart. You are putting the picture of your law into the very physical design and fibre of my heart. You are writing your law on my spirit too. Your finger is writing your love forever onto my heart, and I am only three weeks old.

The Fourth Week—
My Very Significant Blocks

There is something dark and hateful that has been coming near Mother's piece of earth. It is not Love; it is Anti-Love. I do not even want to use Love's name as part of its name when I talk of it. I will call the awful force Evil. Evil is trying to destroy the tablets of my heart where Love's law is written. Evil is planning to destroy me. I can feel it. Mother is restless and anxious. I believe she is beginning to wonder if I am here. I am the size of a very small bean. Love has given me the beginnings of eyes, ears, nose, and all organs.

Mother is stuffing full her big blue suitcase to take home for the vacation period. She seems to like very bright, warm knee socks for under her jeans in this cold time coming up on the winter solstice. She has arranged to ride home in the car of a fellow student along with two additional riders. The car is compact and that keeps her luggage allotment small. She hopes desperately that she won't get nauseous riding in the back seat.

I am developing this week the most amazing set of forty-two or forty-four pairs of dark, square segments all in a row, from my mesoderm tissue. These very significant little blocks are called the protovertebrae or mesoblastic somites. They will grow into not only my vertebrae but also muscle and the under layer of skin. The pairs are arranged in a long, straight row along the line of what will be my head and backbone. Each pair side by side looks like an open book. Now here is what is so amazing, aside from the wonder of Love's creation of me. I am beginning to understand that the forty-two (or four) little block pairs correspond exactly to the words of teaching in books that Love has written somewhere long ago. My body holds during this fourth week a tiny picture of the pattern of those old Love-breathed books. As my body grows older it will retain this picture of the holy books written into its design, but never again will the segmentation be so clearly seen. I think Love wanted to make a living example of His words. If ever there were a perfect human person (I'm not perfect), he could be called the Word made flesh or the living Word. But as an imperfect human, I, too, carry the pattern in my physical make-up.

The somites which Love is making in me have these physiological names: four occipital, eight cervical, twelve thoracic, five lumbar, five sacral, and eight or ten coccygeal. The thirty-three (sometimes thirty-four) vertebrae are from the top downwards seven cervical (neck), twelve thoracic (chest), five lumbar (waist area), five sacral (pelvic area), and four (sometimes five) coccygeal (lowest back). The somites are arranged with five pairs of blocks above the thirty-three pairs that include in their development the thirty-three vertebrae, and four to six pairs below the vertebrae-carrying somites. The thirty-three vertebrae-somites are like a picture of the old holy books given by Love to some people called Jews. The five sacral vertebrae are initially five separate bones that grow together to form one, the sacrum. People don't know why they are named sacral which means sacred; the other bones of the body are generally named from their position or resemblance to some known object. However, Love apparently wanted to give a great big hint that these five bones that become one are a picture of the foundational words Love gave long ago, the first five books given to the Jews, which are the Law.

Above the five sacral vertebrae are the lumbar vertebrae which picture some early books of history. Above them are the twelve thoracic vertebrae, like twelve short books of Love's prophecy, and seven cervical vertebrae to picture seven major books of prophecy, wisdom, and song. Some shorter books are pictured by the coccygeal vertebrae which often grow together to form the coccyx. These books formed the "five rolls" that were read successively on Jewish feast days. I wonder if Mother knows about Love's books. She reads a lot, but nothing written by Love.

The remaining somites, the ones from which no vertebrae develop, picture some newer books that Love has written. The nine of them each represent one of nine authors who wrote down Love's continuing words about two thousand sun-years ago. I surely don't understand why my tiny body should so closely parallel the words Love has written throughout history. Perhaps He really likes this pattern, since He arranged the shape of people and the shape of His words in the same way.

O, Love, how I praise You that You are putting me together to reflect your Holy Book! You saw your finished Book before it was begun; You saw me before I was begun too. Each one of Your books came in its own proper time and sequence; each part of me is developing according to Your design too.

The Fifth Week—Christmas

As the holidays get closer, Mother seems to be fighting off a feeling of dread rather than experiencing the anticipation of former years. This is the first year that she, Joanie, and her mother will be alone together—without her father. He has already sent gifts, mailed from the department store, with very chic, *avant garde* wrappings. He has assured the girls that he will be with them in spirit, but that he and Mother have agreed that he would spend the holidays in the city where he works.

Mother, her mother, and Joanie are all being very cheerful, very busy, and very concerned that this will be a Christmas-as-usual. They are thankful for one another, and each is terribly urgent about wanting to make sure that the other two don't have time to be too sad. Her mother has tickets for *The Nutcracker* ballet, and she and Joanie have planned a brunch for Mother's high school friends home for the holidays. The trivial family traditions built around the tree decorating, the baking, the hanging of stockings, seem to have taken on an additional importance this Christmas. Mother is so happy to be back home in her own room. It hasn't changed a bit. Her not-so-good clothes are waiting unperturbed in her closet for her return. Her old flannel nightgown seems so cozy—the one *no one* would appear in at a college dorm because of its worn and raggedy state. Mother wonders why she feels so unaccountably piqued when she hears that a guest has slept in her room while she is away at college.

Joanie and her mother are curious about why Ben

is not coming around. She tells them that she and Ben have agreed to date others for a while. What she does not tell them is that Ben had been dating others all along while she naively believed that they had an exclusive relationship. The memory of that chance conversation still burns like acid.

"Oh, I know a fellow from your home town over at State," said the girl to Mother in the powder room. "Ben Adamson—he was real serious with a girl in my sorority last year, but they broke up."

"Ben *Adamson*? A tall, slim guy with dark hair who's pre-law?"

"Yeah, that's the one. I'm sure he said he went to high school in your town too. A real bright guy —he's a senior."

The anguish of betrayal covers Mother once more as she thinks about it. She is hurt not so much because he was dating others, although that is hard enough to take, but because of the deceit. He had allowed her to believe that she was his only interest and someday they would be permanently together. Her tears had made Ben uncomfortable, but the only defense he made was to say, "I guess I'm not the monogamous type." Mother has not seen Ben since that confrontation at Thanksgiving.

The problem of where to go for a Christmas service is solved rather neatly. The Cathedral downtown is having a Christmas Eve midnight service open to all comers. Non-members are expressly invited. "Wouldn't it be a wonderful experience to go to the candlelight service at the Cathedral this year?" asks their mother. Joanie and Mother quickly agree. They know that their mother has not gone to their old church yet without their father. There is no way to explain the absence of one's husband on Christmas Eve without announcing the separation.

Perhaps it is the grandeur of the Cathedral in

candlelight, perhaps the magnificence of the choral music, perhaps the crowd of people all gathered to worship, perhaps the unfamiliarity of the liturgy— something is nudging Mother's spirit to wake up. Those are beautiful, old-fashioned words he is speaking: "O God, who hast made this most holy night to shine with the brightness of the true light, grant, we beseech Thee, that, as we have known on earth the mysteries of that Light, we may also come to the fullness of its joys in heaven; through the same Jesus Christ, Thy Son, our Lord, who liveth and reigneth with Thee and the Holy Ghost, ever One God, world without end."

Mother is pondering "the mysteries of that Light." Those words don't mean anything to her. Now he is reading from Isaiah: "Thy people that walked in darkness have seen a great light: they that dwell in the land of the shadow of death, upon them hath the light shined." She doesn't understand that either. ". . . For unto us a child is born, unto us a son is given: and the government shall be upon his shoulder: and his name shall be called Wonderful, Counsellor, The mighty God, The everlasting Father, The Prince of Peace. Of the increase of his government and peace there shall be no end, upon the throne of David, and upon his kingdom, to order it, and to establish it with judgment and with justice from henceforth even for ever. The zeal of the Lord of hosts will perform this."

"So that's where Handel got those words," thinks Mother. "The throne of David" sets her to thinking about Benjamin. She pulls her hurt in around her and doesn't hear any more.

The Sixth Week—The Blood

Before we return to college, Mother is re-arranging her room at home and is making it even more cozy with some new decorator pillows and a downy comforter. She moved some of her little girl things to a bottom drawer, but she doesn't want to part with them yet. She's vacuumed and scrubbed it spotless, washed the mirrors, and straightened all her belongings to perfect order. As we leave, she closes the door firmly and hopes that no one will violate her soft sanctuary while she is away.

I can move myself! My quickening means that enough of my tiny body is together that I can wriggle it. My brain has developed to the extent that my human brain function is measurable by an electroencephalograph. My spirit, which has been the essential part of me from Love from the first, has been given the start of a magnificent brain with which to conceptualize and to express itself. But even if my brain were not too clever, my spirit exists independently and is forever. My spirit praises You, Love, for these new abilities I am discovering. Movement! I didn't know how exciting it would be. My head is quite big compared to the rest of me. That must be to give my magnificent brain plenty of growing room. My shape is becoming more human looking; my arms and legs are started; my eyes are developing lens structure.

My heart is pumping my blood through blood vessels in me now, and I am making my own blood cells. All along my blood has been totally separate from Mother's blood. I am not even her type! I am beginning to perceive that my life is in my blood. I have my own blood, and without a doubt I have life that is sacred to my Creator. The shedding of man's blood must be abhorrent to You, Love. I thank You now for including me in the sum of men whose blood is exceedingly precious to You. How valuable I must be! Though I am only the size of a jewel, I am infinitely more to be treasured, because You must value my blood above all on earth.

I am Yours, my Creator, and You cherish my blood that has Your life. What could man buy me for from You? What non-living product of mine or forest or sea could ever be amassed in sufficient quantity to pay for one drop of my precious living blood? Love, how I love You for making me alive with Your life!

Once again You are teaching me about my life with You, Love, in the way You are designing my blood to function. It is only in You that I can live and move and have my being. My blood pictures what you are to my life. My blood is holy to You, conse- crated by You when You gave me life. It is now set aside in a closed, separated system within me and can- not be contaminated or I may die of blood poisoning. My blood allows for the upbuilding of all my kingdom of tissues that are coming to be and will uphold my body for all of my physical life, as long as You will it.

My blood carries oxygen, like Your life-sustaining breath, wherever it wills in my body; I cannot live without either oxygen or Your breath. My blood car- ries the hormonal messages or instructions that ac- complish Your will for growth, change, or stability in my body. My blood carries daily nourishment to every part of me, as You give it. My blood cleanses every part of me, removing all that is wasted, burned out, or trespassing where it should not be.

My blood maintains the equilibriums of temperature, water, and acidity in my body and resists any temptations to deviate from that which will keep me in perfect health and safety. And my blood fights to deliver me from any evil that would harm me, establishing an astounding network of defenses and aggressive warfare when necessary, even as You protect me from Evil, O my Creator. If damage comes to any part of me, my blood will clot to preserve my life from flowing away from Your purposes. Let me be yours forever, Love.

The Seventh Week—My Face

Mother has begun a vigorous self-improvement campaign—an assault on all fronts. She is watching her diet closely, is doing her calisthenics daily, is drinking extra water, is brushing her hair an extra one hundred strokes each night, and is jogging to class instead of strolling. She has posted a detailed daily schedule on her mirror with time slots for classes, study, library research for term papers *ahead* of due time, relaxation, letter writing, beauty care, and wardrobe attentions. She has saved Friday and Saturday nights for dates and Sunday for dates *only if her studies are current,* as a reward to herself. The schedule tells her what to do next, and she doesn't have to think. She is even more vivacious than her usual bubbly self when with others and has been asked out by two new guys. Right now she's polishing her toenails a bronzy-copper color.

I have a fear and trembling in my parts. What will become my little knees are knocking. My guardian angel is at full alert. Evil is approaching me and desires my life. Evil has a ravenous, urgent, driving compulsion to spill my blood out, because Evil hates Love who has imparted life and blood to me. Evil will try to deceive the people who have power of life or death over me. Evil is concentrating subtle devices on Mother, my earthly father, a Physician, a Nurse, a Social Worker, a Priest, and a Lawgiver. Each one is under deadly assault, because each has a piece of my destiny in his keeping. Though none could create me, each holds the possibility of affirming or negating me, of saving me or killing me. Love holds each one responsible to Him for my blood. He holds the whole land responsible for my blood.

I think the very earth shudders under the defilement of spilled blood.

Much, much more is involved here than my little life, precious as it is to my Creator. The continuance of my land, the blessing of Love on my nation, peace, prosperity, and freedom are somehow all bound up with my life. My land has been fruitful and abundant in its grain and produce until this time. But innocent blood flowing over the land will dwarf its productivity and devastate its promise. My Creator is saying so, and His Word does not fail. Whoever spills my baby blood dries up his own. Oh, Love, do not allow Evil to deceive them, for their own sake, not mine!

I am no longer a faceless person! My face and neck are becoming quite well formed. I wonder who I look like—Mother, Daddy, my grandparents? Nothing seems to be as distinctive in a person as his face. Will mine be beautiful like Mother's or strong like Daddy's? If they could see my becoming face I know that they would love me, because I am stamped with their likeness in my features, and a man surely must love his own flesh.

My highest pleasure in this place is for Love's face to shine upon me. Then by the light of His face, my face may grow to reflect His glory. He has covered me in my mother's womb and His eyes see my substance, yet I am still imperfect. My eyes cannot see You, Love, but I am strangely warmed by Your light. Model my features to give back Your glory. Lift up Your countenance upon my face, Love, and make me a mirror of Your beauty.

Yes, Love, now that I have a face, You know me face to face, even though I must wait to see Your face. You say you have a friend with whom You spoke face to face when he lived on the earth. After You spoke with him the skin on his face was shiny. He had to wear a veil between his face and the people because they were afraid. But when the friend spoke with You again, he took off the veil. There is a heavy veil of flesh between my face and my people now, and they cannot see my new face. But, Love, tell me, is *my* face shiny?

Thank You, Love, for looking on my yet imperfect face with Your holy countenance. Now I am knowing Your peace. I do not have all my capacity to understand yet, but this, Your peace, is beyond understanding anyway.

The Eighth Week—
My Hand and My Bone

Fingers and toes have I! In fact, if something were placed in the palm of my hand, I would grasp it and hold on tight. The amazing potential dexterity of my hands is a sign to me that I, too, may be able to create someday, like Love does. A hand must be a picture of Your sovereign power over all, my Creator. Now that my little hand can do special movements, maybe someday I will be equipped by You to exercise power and authority over Your creation for You. I am especially fascinated by my thumbs, I have a feeling that they are made for some very satisfying purpose.

Mother went to a meeting of a group on campus called the Philosophers' Club, but she was so bored she almost fell asleep. "Even Chess Club would be more interesting than that group!" she is telling her roommate. "I don't know how a person could learn anything about living life there."

My heartbeat is strong now. My people could hear it with instruments or even record it on an electrocardiogram. If somehow my oxygen supply from Mother would stop, I would make gasping movements, even though I have never breathed air. I am about the size of a jelly bean. If someone touched me in here I would bend my neck and move my body. With strong provocation I will move my arms and legs. I have learned to swim with a natural swimmer's stroke! I hope I don't forget how.

My bones are being formed. There is a beautiful

mystery about my bones that I cannot fathom.

My bones have been preformed in membrane and cartilege. Now the long process of ossification has begun. Minerals are gathering in place to gradually harden my bones. My bones will continue to harden all my life; they will gradually become more brittle, less bending, less flexible, more likely to fracture. Gathering from what goes on in this college world, I think people can in the same way harden their spirits against Love over the years of their lives too. Let it never be in my life, my Creator! I love You. Now my spirit, like my unhardened bones, is totally responsive to Your Spirit; my bones are just beginning to calcify, and my spirit is soft, pliable, and available to Love. The cartilege that is preforming most of my skeletal structure is called hyaline cartilege. Hyaline means "glassy"; my first cartilege is clear and translucent in appearance. That's the way I want my spirit to remain, Love; let Your light always shine right through me.

My bones are yet too undeveloped to make blood cells in their marrow; that will begin in my fifth month. However, I have a feeling in my bones that might be called intuition. That intuition is like a knowing activity of my spirit quite apart from my mind, which is yet to be developed. The bones of a man must become sacred by the presence of his spirit and must still be honored even after the spirit of the man has left the body. I think that Love must want bones left behind by the spirit to be put in the earth.

In an incomprehensible way, my bones are picturing the positive commands of the law of Love. I think my bones probably correspond, one on one, with the laws that Love gave through his friend with the shiny face. If One came who perfectly kept the law, no bone of His could be broken. I know that the two

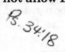

34

large bones that will make up my pelvic girdle will be called "nameless bones" when I am older. Now they are each developing as three bones that will later join into one; the "nameless bone" on each side will attach to the sacrum. These two bones will bear the weight of my upper torso and head, and from them will hang my lower extremities. As these "nameless bones" are developing, I am wanting to love my Creator with all my heart, and with all my soul, and with all my mind, and I am wanting to love other people like I love myself. You are showing me, Love, that my bones, like the laws You give, would be dead and dry unless Your Spirit blows across them and enters them.

Somehow my spirit is intertwined with these new bones. The words Love speaks to me are alive and powerful and very sharp; I feel them in the place of my joints and marrow-to-be. He is saying to me, "I am near them that are of a broken heart; and I save those with a contrite spirit. . . . I keep all their bones: not one of them is broken." Love, please, do not allow Evil to come near my new bones.

Ps. 34:18

The Ninth Week—The Physician

Mother has been denying to herself that I am here, but today she went to visit the Physician. He confirmed to her that I am indeed alive and growing. He asked her gently about my daddy, about her parents, about her school, about her finances, about her goals in life, and about her feelings for me. Mother cried a lot and said she didn't know right now about any of those things. She says she can't marry Daddy. She hasn't told her parents about me. She tells the Physician that they are separated but still married for tax purposes, and she lives with her mother only when she is not at school. She wants to finish her schooling but has no definite purpose for her life. Her father has enough money to "handle" anything. She says she can't feel emotion for me—love or anger. She says her feelings are numb.

Mother asks the Physician if he will "take care of the problem." The Physician looks very serious and sad when he answers. Mother does not know that the Physician has just returned from lunch with two distinguished colleagues. I would not know either if I could not hear the angels talking. Apparently Mother doesn't hear angels when they speak. The other doctors had urged him to join them in a new and probably very profitable venture—an abortion clinic, totally antiseptic, totally equipped for second trimester procedures, totally professional, totally new in this geographic area and, therefore, sure to succeed. They had planned for two doctors at first, but now they need additional funds quickly because the clinic is almost ready to open. They can foresee plenty of work for three or more practitioners. They propose a three-way split after expenses; work by appointment only; and every third week off for skiing, consultation, teaching at the med school, private office practice, or whatever. Overhead and depreciation on the clinic and equipment will make a nice tax write-off. The Physician's current practice is steady but is not growing rapidly because of the declining birth rate.

The Physician is feeling very uncomfortable deep within, for Love is speaking to him through words he memorized as a boy, "My son, if sinners entice thee, consent thou not. If they say, Come with us, let us lay wait for blood, let us lurk privily for the innocent without cause: let us swallow them up alive as the grave; and the whole as those that go down into the pit: we shall find all precious substance, we shall fill our houses with spoil: cast in thy lot among us; let us all have one purse: my son, walk not thou in the way with them; refrain thy foot from their path: for their feet run to evil, and make haste to shed blood. Surely in vain the net is spread in the sight of any bird. And they lay wait for their own blood; they lurk privily for their own lives." He shakes his head as though to shake out the memory of those words.

The Physician is a moral man. He has invested all of his adult life to saving lives and bringing squalling kids into the world. He chose obstetrics-gynecology because of his fascination with life, not pathology and death. But he has compassion for Mother, too. She reminds him of his own daughter. She is too distraught to make a decision now. He fingers a card in his desk drawer. She could fly to the Family Planning Clinic . . . but he has seen some of the psychological trauma that is the aftermath of that place. She is still first trimester. His two very skillful com-

Prov. 1:10

panions will have the local clinic open in a month, with or without him.

The Physician passes Mother the tissue box and tells her that everything is going to be all right. He suggests that she might want to talk with someone at the Community Mental Health Center before she makes any decision. He gives her the name of a social worker there who seems to have her head on straight. He wants to see Mother again in *absolutely no more than three weeks*. He goes to a cabinet and takes out a pile of small boxes, samples of a prenatal vitamin and mineral supplement, and gives them to Mother who stuffs them into her purse. He walks with Mother to the door and puts a fatherly arm on her shoulder.

The Physician is thinking how simple the practice of medicine would be if he could believe that his job was merely the maintenance of biological organisms. But even then, was not the fetus a separate biological organism? What responsibility does he have towards sustaining its life? Why is he, of all his colleagues, disturbed by ethical questions that apparently never enter their consciousnesses? He decides that it is his religious upbringing. He cannot escape it, even though he is not an active church member. He wishes that he were free of moral conviction . . . and yet . . . and yet . . .

The Tenth Week—My Information

The basic structure of my human body is completely formed. I weigh one ounce. I am about as big as a small tangerine section. My head seems less prominent as my body grows and my limbs get longer. I can move specific parts of my body without moving me all over. I have been called "fetus" for a couple of weeks now. Which reminds me, my tiny feet with tiny toes are about as big as two apple seeds, but yet are perfectly shaped. My tongue and lips would respond to a touch, if I got one.

The Physician, Mother, and others are not really thinking of me yet as a *person*. They seem to have a fixed idea of how large a body must be before it assumes personhood. Their limited vision of the universe makes them think that anything less than approximately three or four pounds cannot possibly be a human person. I've decided they don't see angels or other spirits, and they seem equally oblivious to the knowledge that the *spirit* is the essential, eternal part of a person, and the state of a person's body is—well—immaterial. I wonder if I will lose my ability to see and hear the angels after I'm born into the world.

Love is showing me some of His perspective on size which makes the difference between my body and that of a human adult an almost meaningless distinction. The whole world—so big to man's perspective—is but a cosmic speck of dust from Love's view that encompasses the galaxies which are billions of light years in distance from end to end. And yet— the greatest of all miracles is this—Love cares for every molecule and atom of me, made to His specifications and destined to rule this enormous universe with Him. I will never comprehend with my mind what He is revealing to my spirit: size is no indication of value. I do not eagerly anticipate the development of my mind and reasoning power, for I perceive that those faculties will constrict my cosmic vision, and I, too, might begin foolishly to evaluate human life by sizes.

I've heard the angels discussing how the endless, magnificent, all-powerful Creator desired to obliterate forever evaluation by physical size when He conceived the unthinkable, the idea that surprised and startled all the angelic beings, the Incarnation. They whispered that if He, eternal Spirit that cannot be comprehended by any physical limits, chose to limit himself for a time within the confines of one human body, then the human spirit, also eternal but a created thing, can be held in a cell or two. That transcendent concept of the Incarnation reduces to gibberish any feeble attempt to declare that the human spirit, or the breath of the Creator, enters the human tissues at any given point of development after conception or at birth. If Love is able to materialize the preexistent Messiah in a moment of time by the overshadowing of the Holy Spirit, He is also able to create human life in the instant of conception. That means to me that I am fully human now and have been fully human for ten weeks of earthly time.

The earth was void and without form until the Spirit moved across the waters: Spirit preceded form and caused form to develop. In the same way, my form needs the Spirit to assume its shape. In fact, I hear Love personally modeled the form of the first man in His own image from the clay and then breathed life into his lungs.

For Love to speak His intention is for it to be

accomplished. Those scientifically minded people who have studied how humans grow from the seed that becomes alive (like I did) know that each advance and cell specialization is *written in* somehow into the first cells. Development is preformed, mysteriously, accurately, gracefully. That preformation, that compelling pattern, is the activity of the Spirit, which no man can see nor measure. My Creator is the Inventor of chemistry, and He has used His elements in intricate combinations to carry His will through my genes and to conform me to His preconceived idea of me. Genes are like angels since both are messengers from Love's Spirit to effect His will. Ultimately, my Creator is the Organizer and Evoker of my development as a human person. At just the right time, my Organizer tells each new structure and organ to develop. I am created from the smallest of beginnings by the genetic *information* imparted by His Spirit.

But just as some of the angels rebelled against Love and have fallen from His holy purpose for them, some genes go amok too. Love must permit them to wreak havoc as the legal consequence of the sin of our forefathers. However, when that person called the Redeemer comes onto the scene of devastation, He will build from it a spiritual person of great strength; from the old waste places He will raise up the foundations of many generations. He will be called "the repairer of the breach" and "the restorer of paths to dwell in." *ISA 58:12*

The Eleventh Week—Trinity

I am overwhelmed with awe and amazement at what Love is telling me. Now that my parts are differentiated, I can see what has happened in me. I know now that I am made to image Love in His three Persons. But I did not know that the picture of His three functioning personalities was being built right into my cells from my third week of life! My self began to show three germ layers at that time, the ectoderm, the endoderm, and the mesoderm. My little body formed first the ectoderm, then the endoderm, and finally, proceeding and migrating from the ectoderm, the mesoderm. But look closely at what has come in me from each of those three germ layers!

The ectoderm or first layer is developing into my epidermis (outer layer of skin): hair, nails, the linings of my mouth and nose, the lens, retina, and optic nerve of my eyes, the sensory parts of my nose and ears, the enamel-making organs of my teeth, the control-center pituitary gland, my brain, spinal cord, and all the rest of my central and peripheral nervous systems, plus more. Four of my five senses—seeing, hearing, smelling, touching—result from the specially developed cells of my ectoderm layer. All of my thinking, planning, perceiving, feeling of sensation, my internal hormonal timing, and my outside appearance depend on the development of the ectoderm germ layer.

I've learned that the first person is named Father. Father is the Planner and Perceiver of the universe. He is its covering, for in Him we live and move and have our being. He covers himself with light as with a garment. His friend's skin that shone was a reflection of that light from Father. My skin is a picture of Father's protection and containment of me and of all things, and a picture of His visible surface activity in all the world. Father is the Executive Timer, setting the times and seasons for all things in the universe and my pituitary gland is my executive timer for my development, growth, and sustenance. At least four of my five senses will reflect Father's perceptions and will instruct me in how to relate to Him. Father *hears* the cry of the widow or the fatherless child; He *sees* the blood on the houses of His people and passes over them when He smites Egypt; He *smells* a sweet savour from a burnt sacrifice; He puts forth His hand to *touch*. Father warns His people that if we leave Him we will serve gods that are the work of men's hands "which [gods] neither see, nor hear, nor eat, nor smell." The Perfect Son said of our Father that the Son did nothing on His own; He received all of His instructions from His Father. My developing brain and nerves picture the thinking and communicating to His universe of Father.

The second layer, my endoderm, is becoming the linings of my digestive tract—including stomach, my taste mechanisms, intestines, and the secreting parts of my liver, pancreas, thyroid, parathyroid, thymus, and many other glands. The endoderm lines my voice box, windpipe, bronchial tubes, eustachian tubes, middle ear cavity, inner ear drum, mastoid air cells, lungs, bladder, urethra, and more. My reproductive cells are of endoderm origin. My functions of hearing, digesting, breathing, speaking, and reproducing are tied up with my endoderm cells.

My endoderm layer is beginning to picture the working of Love's Holy Spirit—another name of His—in the universe. It is He that oversees the eating of the Word, the digestion of the Word, the absorption of the nutrients of the Word. It is the Holy Spirit that speaks the Word to the world, through the mouths of men, and it is He that is called Breath to me. In fact, He might bypass my brain altogether to speak through me if He wished. He it is that permits my ears to really hear the Word. It is He that will eliminate the impure from me. And it is the Holy Spirit that reproduces for the Kingdom and will cause me to be born again when I hear and receive His Word.

The third layer, my mesoderm germ layer, is building up into all my connective tissues, cartilege and bone, dentine, muscle, blood vessels, lymph glands and vessels, spleen, fat cells, blood cells, the lubrication holding membranes of the joints and bursae, plus more. My framework, my movement, and my circulation are dependent on this layer. My flesh and blood are from my mesoderm layer.

My mesoderm germ layer that is becoming my bone and flesh and blood is picturing the Perfect Son who became flesh. The Son is the name of the other personality of Love. His flesh and blood are to be food to me. My life is sustained by the blood. And the Son is the One who knits me together by joints and ligaments with the increase of Love. The bones picture His perfect fulfillment of the Word of God. Of course, none of my parts work independently of the others. All are part of one indivisible whole. Yet each kind is distinct in its functioning.

Can you see it? Can you see it as I do? When my Creator made me He put pictures of His three personalities into my design. I am trinitarian to the very core of my being. I am made from the first in the image of Love.

The Twelfth Week—The Social Worker

Mother is keeping her appointment at the Community Mental Health Center today. The social worker that the Physician mentioned is out of town this week, but Mother was told that the other social worker would be glad to talk with her. The Social Worker is bigger than Mother physically, and that seems to make Mother even more uncomfortable, since she already has a deep sense of being the troubled one seeking advice. However, the Social Worker is coming around from behind her desk to take a lounge chair near Mother, and that seems to make her less imposing. She offers Mother a Coke, but Mother doesn't think she could handle the drinking of the Coke and the effort of talking about me at the same time. The Social Worker asks Mother a lot of questions, and Mother is talking quite a bit. She is not crying today.

The Social Worker keeps asking Mother about *her* father and about my daddy. She seems to be implying that I am their fault. I didn't know that I was anyone's fault; I hoped I might be someone's glory. Somehow the Social Worker seems to be feeling protective towards Mother and would like to guard her from exploitation from uncaring men. She does seem to like Mother, but then Mother has a winsome and charming way about her even when she is scared and troubled. Thank you, Heavenly Father, for giving me to such a lovable mother!

The Social Worker is consciously adjusting her professional stance to project a warm, caring attitude without appearing too involved or directive. At gut level, the Social Worker is exceedingly angry at

Mother's father, whom she pegs as a deserting father and a mercenary man who did not provide Mother with appropriate male parenting at the crucial stages of her psychological development. The Social Worker knows the type well; her own father was like that. But the issue for right now is to help Mother avoid the trap that has been laid for her, to help her to regain control of her own destiny despite this intrusion on her body and emotional space.

Despite the Social Worker's personal feelings about this case, she values self-determination as the highest good, and she prides herself on raising the consciousness of her clients to as high a level of enlightened self-determination as they are capable of achieving. She begins to discuss viable options with Mother. Only two of them are viable as far as I am concerned—keeping me herself (which is impractical, they both agree), or giving me to a husband and wife who want very much to have a baby in their home. The other options are all death, by various means. The Social Worker seems to have no idea of me as a person; she calls me "it." Mother does think of me as a person now and calls me "the baby." If she would only say "my baby" I would know that she was beginning to love me.

Mother finally says, "I wonder if that wouldn't be murder."

The Social Worker looks a bit perplexed and says, "I didn't think you had strong religious convictions from what you had told me, but . . ."

Mother interrupts with a wry little laugh, "I guess it's obvious I don't have very *strong* religious convictions, but I am concerned with what God would say about this."

The Social Worker is mentally regrouping. At Mother's age she knew God, she thought, but she had moved on to other things. God had not done much for her, and as she advanced in college and graduate school and her professional life, she had become wiser and more concerned with the concrete world. The most important consideration is that this girl reach her full potential; she is obviously intelligent. But self-determination is the first principle; therefore the girl cannot be unduly influenced away from her current feelings at this point. "We don't want you to make a decision that might make you uncomfortable later on, so you ought to think some about the options open to you which we have discussed. Also it might be helpful to you to talk it over with your clergyperson, if you have one. We have a chaplain on the staff if you don't have one here. Perhaps you'd feel better about it afterwards if you at least talked it over with your parents."

Mother says she will talk with the chaplain at her school and think about talking with her mother and father. The Social Worker asks Mother to call her secretary when she is ready with her decision, and she will help with the arrangements, or to call even if she just wants to talk some more. She will always be available to Mother—even at night if Mother suddenly needs to talk. She gives Mother her home number on the back of a little card.

I am glad that people like Mother, but I sense that Evil is controlling the Social Worker, even though she is sincerely trying to help. She seems oblivious to the power of Evil at work. But my guardian angel did not speak to the spirits influencing her.

The Thirteenth Week—The Spy

If there were some way for Mother to see me now, I feel certain that she would love me. I am two ounces heavy already! All of my organ systems are functioning. From now on I'll get bigger, stronger, and more mature, but I don't need anything new from Love; He has formed all the parts of me now. My head is still rather big—about one-third of my total length. I have a high, intellectual-looking forehead. This is the time that my brain cells are growing and multiplying rapidly. I've had my ears lowered, as my growth has continued, and now they are even with my lower jaw. I also appear slimmer in the middle, and I've "sucked in my gut." I had a tiny hernia that I hadn't mentioned, but I've pulled it in from the umbilical cord that attached me to Mother. My eyelids have been growing fast and are now fused at the edges. I have a mustache! Well ... a few fine "vibrissal" hairs on my upper lip, anyway. But that does not mean I am a boy. I'm also getting a few eyebrow hairs and some on my arms and legs. My fingers and toes are well formed, and I have some soft fingernails.

But just listen to all of the things I can do! I can breathe and move my rib cage. Of course, I breathe fluid in this place. I can swallow, digest, urinate, and make tiny, liquid bowel movements. I can taste. In fact, if my amniotic fluid were sweetened I would swallow more often (I like sweets), but if it were made more sour I would quit swallowing. I will respond to strong light or sound by moving my whole self. I can also feel pain. I can learn things. In fact, even my heart will respond to stimulation from my brain by changing its rate of beating. And (maybe I shouldn't tell you this), I like to suck my thumb. I've also discovered this cozy position of curling up.

Since my brain is having its growing heyday these weeks, I'll share some curious facts about my early development. Most of my cells have an uncanny, built-in sense of what they are to be and where they are to go in me. Love tells them by His gene messengers. My nerve cells are particularly clever; they could be transported to a glass tube and they still would grow nerve networks even if my body were not with them any longer. Of course, they would not live long without the rest of me. But they know what they are supposed to do all by themselves. Also, if my hand, for instance, got moved away (but not too far) from where it is supposed to be on my body, the nerve cells that Love sent to ennervate my hand would grow to where it had moved. However, if my hand moved a further distance, other nerve cells in the neighborhood would take up the job of supplying nerves. The cells are not rigidly programmed; they can adapt to new needs. My Creator has given the cells the capacity to change their plans if necessary. In fact, as I was developing, Love straightened out an irregularity or two in me to make me normal.

But there is something that makes me very sad, and I would be afraid if I did not know Love. Parts of me are dying. Yes, some of my dawn-of-creation, fresh, youthful cells have already met with Death. There seems to be an anti-development principle, a force that works *against* my new life, an angry, defiant, hateful push to destroy me *within my own cells*! I know that this death force is a companion of Evil. But how did it get here *inside* me? My blood has special cells called phagocytes that must do the heavy work of dealing with the dead remains of my cells that have already died. Death seems to have a grip on me even before I am born. I feel that I need a special kind of bath to release me from this insidious anti-purpose that breaks out in my own body. While my wonderful little body is expanding to my full potential, something sinister is seeking to ruin and kill me. I knew that Evil was trying to get to me from without, but I am horrified and chagrined to discover that Evil has an agent, an active spy, living right inside this obscure place with me.

The Fourteenth Week—
The Lawgiver

Mother was called by her father on the telephone tonight. He lives in a far city where he works to bring fair and just law to the people. He sounded tired at first, but he brightened as he heard Mother's sweet voice.

"Hello, Baby. I hadn't heard from you in four or five weeks, so I was wondering how you are. Did you get so busy studying that you forgot to call your old, hard-working papa?"

"Oh, hi, Daddy! I'm sorry. I tried once but your secretary was gone and I didn't give my name to the girl who said you were out of town. I'm okay. My classes this term are *tons* of work. I went to the big play-off game last weekend and rooted for your team."

"Didn't seem to help much, Honey, but thanks for your loyalty. I was thinking of coming to surprise you, but we're in the midst of a crisis, as usual, and I couldn't get away."

"What's the crisis, Daddy? Are you still working on environmental standards?"

"That too, Baby. But this one is medical care again—government funding for abortions, actually."

"Oh, yeah? How do you feel about that, Daddy?"

"Well, you know I'm a fiscal conservative in many ways, but my heart gets in the way when it comes to stuff like providing top-notch medical care to the poor and elderly. If we've got it for other expenditures, I think equalizing health care is a first priority. They are having the budget hearings now, and you should hear all the heated rhetoric!"

"No, Daddy, I mean what do you think about *abortion*?"

"Abortion? Do you mean should we fund them for the poor?"

"No, Daddy, I mean are they right or wrong?"

Her father paused for a long silence. The telephone lines were making faint clickings and beepings that weren't noticeable before. "I just don't know, Baby. I haven't thought about it much that way. I more or less assumed that would be the individual's decision. What do *you* think?"

"I don't know either, Daddy. That's why I was asking you. We were discussing it in our Social Problems class."

"I'll think about it some more, Baby, and let you know. We don't think in terms of black and white, right or wrong, much anymore, do we? Everything is in various shades of gray—like my hair, for instance. If you forget to call me again, I'll be totally gray next time you see me!"

"Okay, Daddy. I won't forget. Don't you forget that Joanie's birthday is next week. I sent her a record."

"Sounds loud and raucous. I won't forget her birthday."

"Oh, Daddy! You haven't even heard it! It's by a new group—Retribution—and it's real neat."

"I'm sure Retribution is amply earning theirs. How's your money supply?"

"My money's okay, Dad. I'll probably need more around the first of May, and then a ticket to get home on."

"I'll put that in with my other big bills. Are you going to get a ride home with someone or fly? Oh . . . you said a ticket, you must be planning to fly."

"I'll see, Dad. I'm not going to take home too much junk—just my summer clothes. Uh . . . Dad, I have a friend who might need a loan of about three or four hundred dollars—I'm not sure yet. If she needs it to get through, do you think you could send it?"

"Sure, Baby. If she's a friend of yours, she can have all my money, if there's any left after Joanie's birthday."

"Thanks, Daddy. I love you. Please don't work too hard and try to get some golf in."

"In *this* weather? Well, it should be clearing up shortly. I love you too, Baby. Take care of yourself and *call me.*"

"Okay, Daddy, I will. 'Bye, 'bye."

" 'Bye, Honey."

When Mother hung up the phone she burst into tears. I sure can feel it in here when Mother gets distressed. He calls her "Baby." I'm relieved that Mother has someone who loves her. That means that she knows how to give love. There is hope that she might love me.

The Fifteenth Week—
The Prospectus

I've got reflexes and I've got rhythm! I like to repeat certain movements. But I am not really ready to dance yet; my toes are still spread out like a fan. My arms are now the proper length to match the rest of my body and will stay proportional as I grow. I also have "lanugo"—that's a fine hair that is now growing on my head and body, even eyebrows. My eyes and ears and nose and mouth all have achieved their proper look. In fact, I look properly "human" in all parts of me.

Two important on-going processes have begun in me. My liver has begun to make glycogen. The day that I will be born (if Evil doesn't get me) I will have stored up two or three times the amount of glycogen in an adult's liver. But after only two or three hours of life outside, that glycogen level will have fallen to about one-twentieth of what it was. The stored-up glycogen will keep my blood sugar level at an even rate until my digestive system gets underway with outside food. Love has planned that I won't be hungry for even a few hours when I arrive in the sunlight. The other new process that has begun is the coating of my nerve fibres with myelin to form protective sheaths. This process will go on until I am three years old! As each tract of nerve fibres is completely myelinated, I will be able to do a new function. For instance, I will be able to control my bladder when those nerve fibres are totally sheathed when I am about two years old. I hope I live to learn all the things Love is preparing me for.

Even though I get predigested nourishment from Mother, my stomach and intestines are getting ready for their part in my possible future. My tummy is making enzymes, though it will be a long time until my first meal. My gut is practicing its peristaltic shuffle with anticipation. I surely hope that they won't be disappointed.

But I get cheerful when my spirit remembers my Heavenly Father's power and His purpose in creating me. Death may be a wolf nipping at my heels, snatching some of my cells already, but the Life that is creating me is infinitely stronger. My Father has planned that someone will love me and care for me for a long time out there in the sunshine. He is confident that I can be utterly dependent on someone's nurturing love and protection for many years while He continues my growth physically, mentally, and spiritually. My glycogen supply need only last for the first few hours out there because Love intends that someone will hold me eagerly to her breast to feed me. My nerve fibres may take a leisurely three years to become fully sheathed and functional because He is preparing someone to cherish me in those helpless months. My tummy and intestines already know that Love will open His hand to provide food for them to receive and digest. He will provide my feasts through other people.

I am awed that my future is an assumption inherent in my physical makeup. My body is *anticipating* what Love has planned for me several months, even years, yet to come. All of my life so far seems impelled by some great purpose, some reason toward which I am inexorably attracted, some goal that draws my very being to aim towards it, some glorious end that forms all my beginnings. The very definition of excitement is the responsiveness of my every cell to the urgings of that beautiful possibility in my forever future. O Love, may I never lose that directional signal from You, for if I did, I would be hopelessly lost.

Meanwhile, it is evident that the Father is using even death in me to accomplish His creative work. A number of transient structures appeared in my early days that have since been reabsorbed. The death of some of my cells has contributed in the closing of some tubes, the formation of some vessels, and the remodelling of some of my cartilege and bone—all procedures that are necessary to perfect me. Death is apparently a constant reality of my life, yet the Father uses even that, as He is far mightier, but I sense that He hates Death. Perhaps there could be some way, someone, who could conquer Death and satisfy my heart and the heart of the Father.

The Sixteenth Week—
The Chaplain

Today Mother felt me move. She was having a conversation over coffee and doughnuts with a friend in the snack bar at her ten o'clock break between classes. She kept right on talking, but her heart started pounding rapidly. This afternoon she went to see the college chaplain in his office.

"Thank you for seeing me today," begins Mother. "I know I haven't been very involved in the religious life around here. I'll get right to the point. Is it wrong to have an abortion?"

"Is this an academic question or do you have a personal interest?" responds the chaplain. He likes Mother's directness. Everybody likes my Mother. The chaplain is wearing a green turtleneck and plaid slacks.

"I have a personal interest."

"In that case it depends a lot on your own feelings and circumstances. Do you have a good relationship with the baby's father?"

"No. He's from my hometown but is going to the university in this state instead of at home. We agreed to break up before . . . before I knew. There's no possibility. I don't want him to know . . . ever."

The chaplain asks more questions—the same ones that the Social Worker had asked. In fact, the chaplain had benefited by a year's intensive training in psychological counseling, followed by a year's internship as a special counselor at a large institution. He is as good for Mother as any professional mental

health person. He is very smooth and verbally accomplished and warm and caring besides. The chaplain had left the parish ministry after his divorce,
as it seemed to have an unsettling effect on his
congregation. He likes the campus ministry. It keeps
him young and contemporary. He likes the constant
interplay of ideas, the exposure to the arts, and,
yes, the status it gives him among his peers. He likes
being able to influence the lives of young people
like Mother while they are still open to his sugges-
tions.

The chaplain is more directive in his counseling
than the Social Worker. He feels that a student
coming to him actually wants a moral pronouncement
from the Priest, and the seeker would not be satis-
fied without a definitive word. He also feels uniquely
qualified to give some moral guidance in Mother's
case, because he had helped his ex-wife through the
abortion of their third, unwanted, child. Economically
another baby was unfeasible for them. Of course,
there was the added burden of guilt caused by the
illegality of the abortion. But he had helped her to
see that God affirmed the rights of the individual
above all other considerations—salvation was the
major Christian motif.

"From what you've told me, I think it would be
in your best interest to go ahead and have the abortion—and quickly. You don't want the child. You
don't need the embarrassment of an evident pregnancy. You risk estranging your parents even more from
one another and from you while you still need their
financial and emotional support. You risk bad
publicity for your father. You seem emotionally
strong enough that this shouldn't give you any problems, and you don't have any ethical hang-ups. God
wants to affirm you as a person. He is only interested
in what will make you happy. We must quit thinking

of God as some kind of harsh judge just waiting for us to step over the line. God is Love, remember."

Mother sighs a great relieved sigh. But immediately something in her spirit checks her. "I didn't say that I don't want the child," she says defensively; "there is just no way I could manage it on my own."

"Of course not," agrees the chaplain with a reassuring smile. "Abortion is the only sensible solution in your case."

Mother feels quite comfortable with the chaplain by now. He reminds her of the ministers that she remembers from her younger days when her dad and mom, she and Joanie still went to church together. Those ministers were articulate and urbane fellows too, even witty. "What does the Bible say about abortion?" Mother asks him.

"The Bible? Nothing specifically. That is, the Bible nowhere says 'thou shalt not abort.' The Bible does indicate that God knows us before our birth, and some people believe that means we are to treat the unborn as though they were real persons. Those who make a moral case against abortion think that the commandment against murder applies."

"Doesn't it?"

The chaplain shrugged. "I prefer to believe that the breath of life comes with the first lungfull of air after birth. Nobody can prove otherwise."

I wonder when this man first turned after Evil. Was he not really called by Love to serve Him when he chose to go to the seminary? Did the seminary corrode his first faith? Did Evil become too attractive for him to bear? Did the people demand a new god from him when they gave him their gold? I grieve as Love must grieve that this minister no longer serves the Living God.

The Seventeenth Week—
The Snares

I think I must be a fatherless child. I know that my Heavenly Father created me, but I have no earthly father to acknowledge me as his own. I think that makes me, in a special way, the responsibility of all just men. Those to whom my Creator has given temporal power are the ones to whom He has entrusted the protection of my life, and they are the ones who must answer, along with Mother, for my life if Evil succeeds in killing me.

I usually sleep through Mother's Social Problems class. Mother is usually half alseep herself. But today I learned some very pertinent facts about my country. For instance, the Law is my guardian and protector. What a relief it is to know that I live in a country that promises equal protection of the Law to all its citizens! What confidence it gives me to learn that my country knows that every created soul should have an equal opportunity for *life*, liberty, and the pursuit of happiness! Each man or woman who can vote, administer, or cancel any part of the law of my land can feel a personal glow of satisfaction that the Law protects my life against Evil.

Apparently the Law came at the first and exists now in all its forms for the express purpose of controlling Evil. Without Evil, man would need no law for protection. The Law must be a great restraint on the power of Evil working through man's lust, selfishness, and ignorance. A great shuddering is coming over me to think what would be if there were no law to protect me—Evil would be free to murder me and millions of other citizens, with scarcely a whimper of protest from the unthinking and the uncaring. I can't seem to stop shaking.

Maybe I am shaking because of what the Social Problems class is discussing. Two snares are being laid for my fatherland, my guardian as a fatherless child. The two snares are pervasive errors in thinking about my death and the death of millions of other baby citizens. They are the same two traps that caught the chaplain and muddled his thought so that he was able to murder his own child.

The first snare is the belief that majority public opinion determines morality. Of course that is not true. The Law stands eternally, even if not a living soul remembers it. Civilizations come and go and respond to or ignore God's Law, but God's Law never changes—and the civilizations go quickly when they depart from God's Law. Public opinion is the fickle measure of a nation's spiritual temperature, but it never determines essential right and wrong. If (God forbid) all the priests and all the judges and all the journalists in my country joined together in unholy consent to murder me, God's Law would still stand. I am a human soul with a right to live, and to kill me is to violate God's intent and Law, despite democratic consent.

The second dangerous snare is evaluating life by money—even astronomical sums of money. Just one drop of my life's blood is infinitely more precious than all the gold on earth. Supposedly rational people are comparing the cost in terms of tax money of aborting babies versus the cost of paying for the mother's delivery and post-partum expenses, as though money costs influenced life or death morality. Impossible. Money is totally unrelated to the issues of abortion unless a man loves money more than life. A man cannot love both God and money. A man could not follow God's mandate to protect and care for the fatherless while weighing the financial cost of our care, either at birth or later in our life. God is the owner and master over all the silver and gold and other natural resources; He will allow His wealth to flow to that nation that expends His plenty with total, abandoned giving to the genuinely needy. God's supply will make that nation prosper in every way. But if a man or nation exchanges blood for money, God will dry up His resource and allow the stingy, deceived man or nation to perish.

Oh, Father, keep my fatherland from those two bitter snares. Let my people consider deeply, and let them care for me for their own sake.

Mother seems very agitated by the discussion, but she leaves the class feeling that at least she is no more confused than everybody else about the morality of abortion. How I wish that Mother could hear the angels talking!

The Eighteenth Week—
Manslayer

With some trepidation Mother went back to the Social Worker at the mental health center today. She feels that time is running out on her. Her clothes are getting tight. I weigh one-half pound now, but my comfortable water-bed must weigh quite a bit more. Mother had signed up for golf as her physical education class this term, and she is glad that she did because now she can wear her jeans with a flannel shirt for that class too. Two weeks after next is the spring break. Mother wrote to her mother today to tell her that she will not be flying home for the break, since she is planning to go with some friends to the beach in the south. Now she has come back to the Social Worker for some help with the arrangements for my death.

The Social Worker is appalled that Mother waited six crucial weeks before returning for her further counsel. Mother explains rather lamely that she thought it would be easiest to have it done during the vacation period. The Social Worker decides that Mother is definitely ambivalent about proceeding with the abortion and needs help to firm up her decision.

"You have decided that an abortion is the wisest choice for you?" asks the Social Worker.

"Well...yes...I don't seem to *have* any choice," answers Mother.

"You have considered that an abortion would free you to continue in your career preparation and would avoid a confrontation with your parents and would release you from the humiliation of this unwanted pregnancy?"

"Uh . . . yes, all those things," says Mother. "I don't know what else I could do."

"When we talked before we explored the other possibilities and eliminated them as impractical for you." The Social Worker's voice is taking on a very slight edge of impatience. "Did you talk this over with your parents and the chaplain?"

"Well, not really with my father. I did talk to the chaplain and he thinks it's for the best."

"But this is *your* decision. You need to be convinced in your *own* mind that you are making the wisest choice. Did you talk to your mother at all?"

"Uh . . . no. I couldn't talk to my mother."

"You were not able to communicate effectively with your father either, then? You didn't think he would understand or help?"

"Well, Daddy might understand and help, but I don't want to hurt him."

"You are concerned about your father's ego, then, and that is holding you back?"

"No . . . well . . . I don't know. Daddy loves me . . . I guess I don't want him to think I'm a rotten person."

"You are more concerned about your father's opinion of you than about your own future? I can understand your feelings, but we women *must* learn to break free from the emotional domination of our fathers and other men. Only another woman can really understand what is involved in a decision like this."

"Well, you're a woman. What do you think?"

"Do you mean personally?"

"Yes. I mean what do you think as another woman and not just as a social worker."

"I think, personally and not in any kind of official capacity, that you can't let your life be ruined by your father, your boyfriend, or any man. Men have held us down for centuries by all kinds of force—emotional, physical, religious, economic—and have blackmailed us into giving up our own identities by making us pregnant and then leaving us to take care of the children while they go on doing as they please. You can learn a lot from this experience, bad as it may seem to you. You can rise above male domination in this thing and never let yourself fall under again. You still have your youth, your looks, your future ahead. You can decide right now to be your own person and to be whatever you want to be —independent of men. You will look back some day and think this was the luckiest day of your life if you learn from this difficult time to shake loose from the grip of men on your emotional and physical life."

"But I can't even imagine life without men. Maybe I've been brainwashed all my life."

"I'm offering you freedom from your role stereotypes right now. You can keep your body to yourself and never let yourself be used to propagate more little chauvinists to overpopulate the world. You can relate to men as sexless individuals." The Social Worker is getting red-faced. I wonder what it is about Mother that is causing her to lose her professional cool. "After you rid yourself of the nasty leech you can set your mind to assert your own personality and become master of yourself. The sky is the limit for you. You have fantastic potential. You can't let men hold you down."

Mother is turning pale. She does not hate men, and she will not let anyone call me a nasty leech. She was mistaken to come here for help. The Social Worker is the one who needs help. Mother picks up her purse abruptly and leaves the office. The secretary looks up, surprised, as Mother almost runs by her desk.

I think Evil overshot today. The logical arguments sounded right to Mother until the venom began to leak and then spill out. Mother is not seeking hatred. She is seeking Love.

The Nineteenth Week—
The Yearning Motion

All this talk about men and women reminds me that I know definitely now which sex I am. Of course, my sex is written into every cell of my body in my pair of sex-determining chromosomes, so from the first Love intended for me to be distinctly of my gender. But now anyone viewing me from the outside could tell whether I am a girl baby or a boy baby. I am not going to tell which I am, because that is the big mystery question that people like to ponder until my birth, and I don't want to ruin anyone's fun.

The question of my sex is important to everyone because my sex is a qualitative difference of vast significance. Many try to erase the built-in difference by various bizarre behaviors because they think wrongly that one sex is somehow better or more advantaged than the other. When one tries to deny his sexual difference, he loses an essential quality integral to him as a unique and precious creation. Evil wants to make people as sexless as possible, because Evil knows that a spiritual understanding of complementary sexual roles will lead people to seek eternal union with their Lover-Creator. Evil desires that human souls experience eternal separation from their Lover-Creator, just as Evil must endure. If Evil can convince people to deny their true sexuality, they may not even desire eternal spiritual union with God, because they will never experience the joy of a spiritual union here on earth with a beloved mate to whet their appetites and cause a yearning in their souls for a similar but vastly higher eternal bliss. Evil is trying also to destroy the family so that the children already here will be lost and without values or appropriate sex models, and so that no new human souls will be born.

Evil tries to obliterate all sexual difference. Primarily Evil does this by convincing girls that they ought to be just like the guys in dress, interests, behaviors, and especially careers. Evil convinces a few men to emulate feminine behaviors, too, but that is usually in the interest of perverted sexual gratification. Girls are more easily persuaded to adopt male characteristics because maleness is identified with money, and, hence, power and freedom. Money is apparently a god that incites greed equally in the hearts of male and female.

Now my Father is showing me what it means to be male or female. It does *not* mean that I cannot tinker mechanically or cook a gourmet meal if I am the "wrong" sex for that activity. It does mean certain basic differences. If I am a boy I am wonderfully made for heavy global responsibilities, working under pressure, governing, discovering, leading, protecting, building, providing, fighting, and man-style loving. If I am a girl I am especially suited for more local, detailed responsibilities, appreciating, sensitivity to fine distinctions and feelings, beautifying, comforting, following, nurturing, supporting (emotionally), creating, talking, and woman-style loving. Neither male nor female is complete without the other. Either will learn from the other sex and share in some of the activities typical of the other sex, but the *emphasis*, the integrating personality of the person is determined by God to be of one kind or the other.

But these sex-defined activities are largely learned from models of the same sex, usually from parents.

Why not, then, suggests Evil, why not incorporate *all* of the activities into both sexes so that each individual will be a total, well-rounded human being with the broadest possible spectrum of activities? Because all motion would stop, all progress halt, all motivation cease. It is the very polarity of the two kinds, masculine and feminine, the oppositeness, that keeps life moving. The attraction for and the movement towards the opposite sex with the urge for completion in its myriad aspects is the *primum mobile*, the first moving force, that motivates man and woman on earth. That compelling incompleteness is planned by God to instruct us about our own ultimate incompleteness without Him. Without sexual difference that denotes partialness to us we could have no concept of purpose, striving, searching, longing, or movement toward fulfillment. Our difference teaches us to yearn. Once we know to yearn, we can learn that what we ultimately yearn for is God and that our temporal yearning for a sexual completeness is a metaphor designed to show us that pleasantly. Some folk don't need the metaphor in their adult life to seek God; most folk do. The first message of my sexuality is clear: I need someone other than myself to be whole and happy and I must move towards finding him/her. The final message of my sexuality may not be as easily perceived: I need God to complete me for eternal happiness, and He has moved towards me.

Regrettably, I probably won't remember all this after I'm born—if I get born. My spirit will always be as accessible to my Father, but my spirit will not be nearly as accessible to my own consciousness.

I just want to thank You, Father, for making me the sex that I am. From what You have told me, my sex is exactly what I want to be, and the other sex sounds . . . well . . . *interesting*.

The Twentieth Week—
The Prayer

Mother is calling out to God this evening in her own room. She doesn't know God or how to talk with Him, but she has heard about Him and thinks He must exist. She sees the earth and the beauty and complexity of His creation, and somehow she knows in her spirit that God has made it all. She knows that she is gripped by trouble, sorrow, and eventual death that are overwhelming her, but she doesn't know how to escape from them. She feels utterly alone and, despite her attempts at courage, utterly helpless.

"Oh, God, I don't know where You are or who You are, but I need You. I can't go on living by myself. I am totally alone with my problem. Nobody seems to be able to help or to be able to tell me what is the right thing to do. I want to do the right thing, God, but how am I to know what is right and what is wrong? What do *You* want, God? Do You want me to go ahead and make the most I can of myself and never let my family know about this? Do You want me to have an abortion? Is it really okay with You?

"I can't help but feel that my baby is a real person inside me right now. Am I wrong? Is my baby just a hunk of tissue now and not really a person yet? I need to know, God. I don't want to be a murderer. Show me, God.

"And, God, You know I don't hate life. I love little babies and I love men too. I love my daddy and my teachers and my uncles and grandpas and my friends and I love . . . Benji. Why do I feel that I'm being pushed to hate and kill? Please help me, God. Please help me. If You do, I promise to never get involved in this again. And, God. . ."

Mother's prayer is interrupted by the ringing of the telephone. It is her mother, long distance.

"What's the matter, Jill? Your voice sounds funny."

"Nothing, Mom. I think I'm getting a cold."

"Joanie and I really want you to come home next week for your break. Do you want to go to the beach that badly? It's been since Christmas that we've seen you. Anyway, they always have riots and carrying on at the beach during the spring vacation, and I'd rather if you didn't go there with just a bunch of kids."

"Oh, Mother! I'll be fine. I can take care of myself. I already promised."

"Who are you going with?"

"Uh . . . a couple of girls from the dorm and a couple of girls from their sorority. One of them has an aunt who lives down there."

"What's her name? How could we get in touch with you?"

"I'll have to find out and call you back."

"Well, you can't enjoy yourself with a cold anyhow. Why don't you cancel and come home? We'll go to the special exhibit at the art museum, and Joanie wants you to go shopping with her for her prom dress."

"I can't, Mom."

"What do you mean, you 'can't'?"

"I just *can't.*"

"Jill, there's something wrong. You'd better just tell me."

"All right . . . I'll *tell* you what's wrong. I'm four

and a half months pregnant," blurted out Mother. "So that's what's wrong!"

After a pause her mother's voice came cool and deliberate. "Jill, you know what you must do about that. *What have you been waiting for?*"

"I don't know, Mom. I just can't seem to make myself do it."

"Jill, I'm coming out there. I'll just have to miss the state convention. I'll go with you. This is more important."

"No, Mother. *Please* don't come. I've seen a doctor. I'll go back to him right away. I promise. Please don't come."

"Jill, you can't let a thing like this ruin your life. You've *got* to have it taken care of right away. Put it on your father's medical insurance. He'll have to know anyway. If there's any problem with the insurance, let me know and I'll send a check. Don't wait any longer. The longer you wait the more complications can occur. You can rest up next week with no classes and get your strength back."

"All right, Mom."

"Are you sure you don't want me to come out? I can be there tomorrow afternoon."

"I'm sure, Mom. I'd feel better to do this on my own."

"Okay, Darling. Be sure to call me immediately if there's any problem getting it done. And please call me afterwards so I can relax."

"Yes, Mother. Thanks for calling. 'Bye now."

"Good-bye, Jill."

God sure has a funny way about answering prayers. I think Evil must be able to use mothers, too. Is there no remedy to stop Evil? Can Evil have his ugly will to kill me with no resistance? Does no one care for my life?

The Twenty-first Week—
The Arrangements

I was wrong. I didn't understand. The Law in my land does *not* protect me. I should have known —the new abortion clinic, the Social Worker's options, the urgings of the chaplain and my grandmother—they were not for an *illegal* act, just a heinous act. My continued existence is totally at the mercy of Mother.

She is amazed at how quickly she got her appointment with the Physician—the same afternoon that she called. The nurse asked her to bring in a urine specimen in a clean bottle. Mother wondered why the nurse suspected she might use a dirty bottle and laughed a bit. My Mother has not lost her sense of humor. Mother watches the other, happy expectant mothers in the waiting room closely, and she keeps her left hand out of sight.

The Physician is truly concerned to see Mother back again. He had assumed she had gone to the campus clinic or elsewhere many weeks before since she had not returned to talk with him within the three weeks he had mandated. "Where have you been, Jill," he asks gently.

"I've been thinking it over," Mother replies. "I'm a reflective person."

"I should say so," says the Physician drily. "What have you decided?"

"I've decided to go through with it."

"Decided to go through with what? The pregnancy or an abortion?"

"Oh. The abortion." Mother's voice seems very

tiny. "My mother thinks I should."

"What do *you* think?"

"I guess it is for the best." A tear is forming in the corner of each eye, and Mother is struggling to keep her composure.

The Physician can feel the uproar in his own conscience starting up again. Dammit, this is strictly a medical matter. Routine. Yes, it happens every day. She's a pretty, bright child and he's got to help her get through this thing without psychological trauma. Why does he feel so responsible for this one?

"All right. Let's examine you." He calls the nurse in.

The second-trimester clinic isn't open yet. The facilities are ready, but the clinic has not been approved for state funds for the welfare abortion cases, and they can't get it off the ground without those tax dollars. Most second-trimester cases are not among the elite. The poor seem to have a stronger feeling for children—even after several—and often must be psychologically coerced by the practical wisdom of their social workers before considering abortions. The Women's Health Clinic, as it is to be called, will be opening without the Physician's money or presence. He could not bring himself to violate his conscience, wherever it came from, as his way of practice—even for more money and an easier schedule. His colleagues did not really understand his reluctance, although they said they respected his convictions. They found the funds elsewhere but had not yet engaged a third active partner. The Physician was really quite relieved when his wife threw a fit over the prospect of his joining the clinic. Her intense emotion gave his faltering conscience some much-needed support.

"Jill, we're going to have to take you to St.

Luke's Hospital for this. I will do a hysterotomy under general anesthesia—that's like a Caesarian section. Can you check in over there on Sunday afternoon?" Necessary for the mother's health. The hospital administration is not going to be too happy about this, but they will do it. Ninety percent of his deliveries are there.

"Yes. About what time? Will it leave a big scar?"

"Not too awful—like any abdominal surgery. It will be a low scar. You can still wear your bikini. Check in by four-thirty. You'll need some tests, and they will give you a light supper there."

"What shall I bring with me? I mean, do I need nightgowns or what?"

"You'll wear a hospital gown while you are there, but you'll want to bring your own robe and slippers, your toothbrush and comb, your cosmetics. Also you'll need to know your dad's insurance policy company and number, and you'll need some way to pay for the few items not covered by the policy before you leave the hospital."

"Will they charge it to a credit card?"

"Yes. When you get the policy number, phone my nurse too. You should be able to go back to the dorm before the end of the week. Do you have someone who can come to take you back to the dorm?"

"I guess I'll get a cab. I'll be able to walk okay, won't I?"

"Sure. You'll feel *almost* as good as new—a little sore and stiff, and, Jill. . ." He pauses quite awhile.

"Yes, Sir?"

"Don't worry about anything. I'll take good care of you."

My prospects, frankly, are not looking too good. The Physician is not an evil man, but why does he seem unable to stop Evil? He has refused Evil on a large scale, but his genuine compassion for Mother is being used by Evil to destroy me.

The Twenty-second Week—
The Nurse

We are here in the hospital bed. Mother is wearing the new blue robe she bought over the hospital gown because she hates having her backside bare. Tears keep seeping out of her eyes while she is trying to read *The Return of the Native* for her literature class. The other bed in the room is empty. Since the sun is setting, Mother is looking for the light cord. On second thought, maybe she won't read for a while, and she won't turn the light on until those tears stop.

There is a hushed but heated discussion going on at the nurses' station. Mother hadn't expected the nurses to be as cold and uncommunicative as they seem to be here.

"I won't do it," says one blonde nurse. "Get somebody else."

"I will," says the Nurse. "Give them here to me. Do you have a pen?" In a moment the Nurse comes into Mother's room. "Hello, Jill," says the Nurse in a kind voice. "I'm Mrs. Symes. How are you feeling?"

"Okay, thank you," says Mother.

"Jill, we have some papers that the admissions people forgot to complete. We need you to sign a consent to dispose of the dead fetus, and we need some more information for the fetal death certificate."

"For the *what*?"

"The fetal death certificate. The state requires it." I give Mother a good strong kick.

"But . . . but my baby's not dead yet . . . how can I fill out a death certificate?" Mother bursts into tears.

"We know. But these papers giving your consent to its death must be completed before the operation to relieve the hospital of legal responsibility . . ."

"Why do you need a death certificate if my baby is not a real person yet?" sobs Mother. "You don't write up a death certificate for a tumor or a tonsil or an appendix or . . . or . . ."

The Nurse puts down the paper and hands Mother a tissue. "The baby *is* a real person," she says. "You know that too, don't you?"

"Yes," Mother sniffs, "but there's no other way for me. I haven't got what it would take to go through a whole pregnancy. I'm not even married, you know, and I couldn't stand to go to a home for unwed mothers or anything like that."

"Yes, I know, Jill. But there is Someone who can help you through this."

"Someone? Do you mean God? What can He do now?"

"It's nothing from the outside, Jill, but you can come to know Him personally as your Savior and your Friend. If you ask Jesus to take over your life, He will do it, and He'll give you the strength and the courage to do anything that He asks of you."

"Jesus? I believe in Jesus. I mean I know He was the Son of God and all that. I used to go to Sunday school."

"Yes, Jill. But each of us must at one time or another *ask* God for the forgiveness of our sins at the cost of Jesus' blood on the cross. We need to truly turn away from our sins and humble our will before Him. Then we can receive Jesus into our hearts to actually live there *in* us and be the Lord of our lives. He really does move inside with His Holy Spirit, and you will be a new person when He comes."

"I know I have sinned, all right. I feel so dirty. I mean not only because of my sex life, but I must be some kind of a rotten mother to agree to have my baby killed. . . . " Mother can't talk anymore, as she is sobbing again.

The Nurse puts her arms around Mother. "Sin *is* always sad," she says, "but Jesus is stronger than sin, stronger than Evil. He is the mighty Son of God, the Redeemer—and He can make something very beautiful out of your life."

"Even now? After I've done this?"

"Even now. He's been waiting for you to call on Him for help. He will wash you as clean as a newborn baby and give you a brand new life. And He will take care of both you and your baby. He loves you as no human person can ever love you."

"I want to receive Him. I want to be forgiven and to be a new person. And I want Him to take care of my baby for me. How do I receive Jesus?"

"Just tell God that you know you have sinned and ask for His forgiveness. Thank Him for Jesus' blood that washes you clean of your sin. Ask Jesus to take over your life and to come to live in your heart. And then thank Him that He has heard your prayer and that you are now His forever."

Mother is doing that with more tears here in the hospital room, and I am leaping for joy in her womb. Evil is defeated. Jesus is the Name of the One who has defeated Evil. Jesus is the One who has rescued both Mother and me from Evil. I can't describe what happened, but a deep peace seemed to come over Mother. I could feel it even here in this obscure place. The Nurse tells Mother that she will call the Physician and cancel the arrangements. Mother should stay overnight at the hospital anyway and she will be discharged in the morning after he comes to see her.

The Nurse promises to pick up Mother in the morning so that she can take her to meet some other Christian people who will help us.

The Twenty-third Week—Forgiveness

Mother is back into her regular class schedule. She has decided with the Physician that since she is feeling fine, she can finish out the semester's work. She just keeps falling asleep when she tries to study on her bed! The Physician got tears in his eyes when Mother told him last Monday at the hospital that she is a new person in Jesus and that she is going to carry me to term. If only he could believe that it was that simple, like when he was a child . . . He didn't trust himself to say anything at all. She will see him at his office every three weeks until school is finished in June.

Mother went with the Nurse on that bright, sunny morning and talked with a counselor at a Christian group that helps pregnant girls to have their babies. The counselor there offered all kinds of help to Mother —clothes, finances, a place to stay later on, practical information about pregnancy and about adoption procedures if she should decide to give me to a family. Mother felt that the counselor really cared about her and about me. She is going to return later on to talk about adoption. Mother never knew that all that help was available for her. The Nurse also introduced Mother to her priest who is a kindly, loving, lively man who also loves Jesus. He told her about a Christian Youth Fellowship that meets on Sunday evenings in a private house near the campus. He said that he would ask a couple of the students to come pick her up for it next Sunday. They were not yet back from the spring break last week.

Mother called her mother, too, that Monday night

and told her what had happened to her and about her decision to bring me to birth. Her mother didn't understand at first and kept telling Mother to get on with it. Finally she decided that Mother had been strongly influenced by some religious people in her time of emotional stress and that she needed time to simmer down. She asked Mother to please go to see a psychiatrist or else come home. Mother said she planned to finish out the school term and agreed to see a psychiatrist. Then she called the priest and asked him for the name of a Christian psychiatrist, and the next day she made an appointment with him.

Maybe in the world's eye Mother does need a psychiatrist. She is filled with joy in the midst of her terrible predicament. If anyone needs a testimonial, *I* can tell him that Mother's whole body changed when Jesus' Spirit moved in. She feels clean, clean, clean at last. She is so thrilled every time I move. "You're alive! Alive, you dear little kid. You'd better be thanking the Lord for that!" I am! I am! And then she says it. "I love you, little kid. I love you just like God loves me. He's going to work it out for you. You'll see. Someday you'll get to know Jesus too."

What is it about forgiveness that fills a person with joy? What is it about forgiveness that makes one affirm life, celebrate life? For the first time Mother feels really honest and open before God and men. She has confessed that darkness in her that she felt she must hide, and with her confession all her heavy guilt disappeared. She is surrounded by God's love—within, without, beneath, above. The Spirit within her is teaching her. She is *sincere*, through and through. There are no longer two Jills, the ideal Jill and the ugly Jill. Now there is only one Jill—Jill the forgiven, Jill the purified, Jill the beloved of God. She feels that light could shine right through her. She feels energized by a new power.

She knows now that when she sins she is instantly forgiven as she confesses to her Father, because of the shed blood of Jesus that applies to her.

Mother has been reading in the New Testament that the priest had given her. He told her to start with the Gospel of John. She is amazed that she can understand it. Before the Bible never made any sense to her. She reads and reads and reads, with the hunger of a lover reading letters from her beloved. She must force herself to do her ordinary college studying.

Mother shared her experience of Jesus with her roommate the first night that she returned from home after the spring break. The roommate is relieved that Mother has found a solution to her problem, for, of course, the roommate knew about me. She is glad that Mother is happy again. She just hopes that Mother is doing the right thing. Mother is rather puzzled that her roommate doesn't want to pray for forgiveness and Jesus immediately too. Jesus didn't just help her with the problem of me—her whole *life* was the problem. Everybody's whole life is the problem before God's forgiveness breaks through.

Mother has to restrain herself from shouting for joy because she is now righteous with the Lord's righteousness, and God no longer sees any sin in her but only Christ's covering. The angels are rejoicing too. They say it will be much later before Mother learns that not everyone has the same kind of exuberant conversion that she has had. My Father seems to know that she needs some extra encouragement because she is quite alone in her everyday situation. That joy is in her heart to stay; it will grow deeper and deeper, though her emotions may fluctuate around it. And, I hear, there are those who would say that a "religious" person should still be weeping with shame and remorse!

The Twenty-fourth Week—The Visit

Today Mother got another phone call from her father. She has carefully remembered to call him for brief chats at his office almost every other week, so she is surprised to hear again so quickly from him.

"Hi, Baby. It's me, your old papa."

"Hi, Daddy! What a surprise!"

"I think you're going to be even more surprised, Honey. I'm right here at your airport. I'm about to rent a car, and I'll be out to see you. I just wanted to check to make sure you were at the dorm. . . . Your mother called me."

"Oh."

"It's all right, Baby. We love you, and I just wanted to talk to you and to see for myself that you are okay. I'll be out in about an hour and we can go out for supper somewhere. Can you get away?"

"Sure, Daddy. I'll be ready."

Mother is rather nervous as she gets dressed. She tries on three different blouses and finally decides on the unbleached muslin with lace. She is glad that she washed her hair this morning. All the while she is praying in stops and starts. "Please help him to understand, Father . . . Give me the right words to say . . . Don't let him be hurt . . . Help me not to look too big . . . Oh, Jesus, just be with me!"

Her father holds her close for a long time when he sees her. Mother is getting sniffly, but gives him a bright smile. "It's not as bad as you might think, Daddy. God has used this to show me some *very important things* about myself and about Him and about life. He has shown me that all people are sinners, including me, but that there is free forgiveness in Jesus. I feel forgiven, Daddy, and this is the best I've ever felt since I was a little girl. And He's shown me that I can be part of His creative plan by bringing this little person safely to life. My little kid will have a chance to grow and to get to know God too. I mean, I'm talking about eternal life, Daddy, not just a few years here. My little kid can have *eternal* life, just like I have."

"I brought you a present," said her father with a smile. He handed her a heavy bookstore paper bag. "It's some black and white for you." Mother opened the bag and took out a thick Bible with study notes.

"Oh, Daddy! How did you know I wanted one so badly? I *need* one with the Old Testament too! Thank you so much!"

"You're welcome, Baby. I just knew."

"Daddy, I just *know* that abortion is wrong. I knew it in my heart before but I couldn't give any reasons why I knew. I felt so frustrated because no one else seemed to know. I'm going to find out what God says about it in His Word. And I want to *show* you that abortion is *always* wrong because it kills a person God has created. I know you want to help the poor women and don't want them butchered in illegal and dirty attempts at abortion. But there has to be a better way than killing the babies. You *can't* give them government money for that, Daddy. That makes all of us murderers. We have to figure out a way to help both the mothers and the babies."

"You look in your Bible, Honey. I'll listen to what you have to say. Just remember that most poor women have a lot of pressures that you don't have to worry about."

"I know, Daddy. I'm grateful to God for providing for me. But God doesn't have one standard for rich, educated people's babies and another for the babies of the poor and uneducated. Money and education don't count at all when we're talking about eternal life. Every single soul must have the opportunity to receive God's forgiveness and to live forever. To kill any baby is horribly wrong. The quality of his potential life on earth is of no consequence. In fact, the babies who have it tough may be the very ones who will turn to God first and get *eternal* life."

"Well, Honey. There's the problem also of getting the funds to those poor women who absolutely need an abortion medically or they will die."

"How many are there who are in that kind of a fix, Daddy?"

"Only a few."

"Would doctors and hospitals refuse to care for those few without government funds?"

"Of course not."

"If the government agrees to pay for any abortion, it is like telling the uneducated woman that baby-murder is okay. It is also telling the private sector that it's morally acceptable to murder the unborn. Daddy, *I almost killed my baby!*"

"All right, Honey. I understand how you feel. Where do you want to go for dinner? And then we'll talk about how we're going to take good care of you and your baby."

The Twenty-fifth Week—Integration

With all the recent excitement and my narrow escape from death, I've neglected to record my physical progress in my journal. I weigh well over a pound now and am increasing in weight rapidly. I am more than halfway to my intended length at birth time. From now on I will grow about five centimeters in length each month. If even God is starting to teach me in metric, I guess we will all have to convert. My legs have been growing in length but they are still shorter than my arms. My teeth have begun to calcify so that I will have hidden pearly-whites when I am born. My fine lanugo hair covers most of my body. My lungs are delineated and their capillary system is now developing. My sebaceous glands are actively secreting some greasy kid stuff called "sebum" on my skin surface. My thyroid gland has been able to synthesize its own hormones for over a month now. I have definite cycles of quiet and movement that Mother can feel.

If Evil had succeeded and I had been aborted by hysterotomy, I would have moved, breathed, and maybe cried in a frantic effort to live. I might have survived if I were born at that age and were helped. Nurses know this and very few will assist with an abortion at my age. Some courageous nurses have risked their jobs by refusing to participate in murder and many have forced hospital administrators to deny their facilities for abortions. Nurses seem to have hearts full of compassion and a deep sense that life is God's prerogative to give or take. In fact, I hear that God's friend with the shiny face was saved from death by a midwife-nurse who obeyed God rather than man at the time of his birth in Egypt long ago.

One of the most amazing things about my body is the exactness of God's design that puts every part into an intricate and precise relationship with every other part at the perfect time. Nothing is superfluous; nothing can exist apart from the whole. We don't understand yet the function of the so-called vestigial organs—the parts of me that *appear* to have no job to do in the human body, the appendix, the ear muscles, and the bones of the coccyx (my tail-end). During my fifth week of life I also grew a tiny tail which later retrogressed and disappeared. We may discover real physical reasons for these organs at a later time, but we can know now that each is at least symbolic of a spiritual lesson. The bones of the coccyx are necessary to spiritually represent four (or five) books of the Scripture in the spinal picture of the Old Testament. The tail that appears and then disappears takes on a startling significance when one considers that God warns that the prophet who teaches lies is the tail. The ear muscles might be what allow a man to "incline his ears" to the Word as God so frequently urges. And it is possible, though not too probable, that the vermiform (literally, "worm-shaped") appendix pictures that abhorrent worm of man that never dies in the unquenchable fire. These few difficult, bestigial exceptions are a very small minority. We can readily see the vital interworkings of nearly every part of the human body, each receiving its "orders" from the head.

The human body is like a picture of the relationships of Christians to one another and to Christ here on earth. Jesus is the Head and various Christians are the members. No member can live long without being integrated into the living body. That is why the Nurse was careful to assure that Mother would be brought into a body of believers to nurture her new life. The body to which she comes will benefit from the life of Christ in her, too. She no doubt has some special function for this time that is needed by the church in this place.

Mother was no stranger to some of the members of the student Christian Fellowship on Sunday nights. She had known some of them casually in classes or from the dining hall. A couple of the girls are from her dorm. But when the group is gathered together for singing praises and Bible study and prayer, Mother finds a tangible Power and Presence that is far more than the sum of the individual parts. Jesus is there in the midst of them. Her spirit unfolds like a flower in the sunshine of love and worship.

The fellows and girls welcomed her as a new sister, and she immediately felt that she is indeed one of them. One of the guys, Roger, has started to pick her up for church on Sunday mornings, too, as it is quite a walk to the church. No one has put her down because of her "condition." Each of them has experienced forgiveness, too, and each is eager to share the wonder of God's grace to them.

I can't help wondering what part of the body Mother is like—what function she will have for the group. I know that body and parts is just picture language, but . . . I think Mother must be the smile.

The Twenty-sixth Week—
The Psychiatrist

Today Mother is keeping her promise and is going to see the Psychiatrist. It seems a lot of trouble to her, as she has to take the bus clear downtown to his office, but she is sure it will be worth it to see a *Christian* psychiatrist. But it is a beautiful May day and the bus windows are open to give her a clear view of the flowers everywhere. She wonders what kind of people will be in his waiting room. No one else is there waiting; apparently he keeps a tightly controlled schedule. The receptionist (is she a nurse or isn't she?) invites her to go in.

"What can I do for you," asks the round-faced, small man with a fuzzy beard, after he introduces himself to Mother.

"I'm just fine," says Mother, "but I promised my mother I'd talk to a psychiatrist, and a friend's priest gave me your name."

"Why does your mother want you to talk to a psychiatrist?"

"She's afraid that I'm crazy because I'm pregnant and don't want an abortion."

"Are you?"

Mother laughed her tinkling laugh. "I think that's what you're supposed to tell *me*."

"Why don't you want the abortion?"

"Because I've become a Christian and I want to give my baby a chance to live. I really think that is what God wants too."

"Have you decided what you will do with the baby after he's born?"

"I think I'll give him or her up for adoption through a Christian adoption agency if they will *promise* me that he or she will go to a home where they will teach him or her about Jesus. I want my baby to have eternal life. I couldn't make a good home for a baby yet."

"How do you feel about yourself these days?"

"I feel increasingly pudgy, but I'm a new person in Christ."

"What do you mean by 'a new person'?"

"I mean my old sins are washed away and God's Spirit is teaching me how to live an entirely new way. I mean I still sin but I don't *want* to now, and I get forgiven right away when I slip up."

"You mean you don't feel guilty about anything?"

"No, Sir. Jesus takes away all my guilt. I'm clean."

"How does God teach you?"

"When I read the Bible, mostly. Sometimes I just *know*."

"Do you ever hear His voice?"

"No . . . not an out loud voice."

"Any voice?"

"No . . . no voices."

"Are you sleeping okay?"

"Yes sir, and I seem to need an afternoon nap, too!"

"How about eating? How's your appetite?"

"I'm hungry most of the time, but I'm trying to use restraint."

"Any thoughts of self-destruction?"

"No . . . before I became a Christian it occurred to me."

"But not since?"

"No way."

"Tell me a bit about your family. How do you feel about them?"

"Well, I just love my parents and my sister. I'm very sad that Mom and Dad are breaking up."

The Psychiatrist asked a number of innocuous questions about her family, her home town, my daddy, her friends, and other ordinary stuff. Mother said she still loved all of her friends, but that her new Christian friends were special in a different way. He seems distracted for a minute and is fooling with his desk calendar. "I seem to be behind on my calendar here . . . What's the date, anyhow?"

"May 11."

"Thanks. Do you like going to college here?"

"Yes. Very much."

"Any problems?"

"Not that I can think of."

"How are your studies?"

"I get good grades."

"Do you have any goal you're working towards?"

"Right now I just want to finish up this term, have my baby next August and help other people to understand that an unborn child is a *real person*. Then I'll think about what God has for me later on."

"Do you think anyone is working against you?"

Mother looked at him blankly. "No, why would they?"

"This must be a little hard on you. Socially, I mean. Do you ever get depressed?"

"I did at first, but not since I've made my decision to accept Jesus into my life and to give my baby life instead of death. If I start to get depressed, I just thank God for all He has done for me."

"Anything else you want to talk about?"

"Uh . . . no. I can't think of anything."

The Psychiatrist stands up. "You seem to be doing fine. Call me if any problems come up." Mother says thank you and good-bye. She is puzzled that he didn't ask her any really deep questions about her past and her parents or give her some kind of a mental test—like ink blots. She gives the receptionist her father's charge card. For that the shrink gets forty dollars! Mother wonders why the Christian Psychiatrist didn't respond to her expression of faith with an enthusiastic expression of his own faith in Jesus. Maybe he just doesn't talk about God on the job. Now she can call her mother and tell her that she has a clean bill of mental health. She wonders if the Christian Psychiatrist is any different in his practice than an ordinary psychiatrist.

The Twenty-seventh Week—Destiny

"Daddy: Just listen to this!" Mother is writing a letter to her father on yellow paper with daisies instead of phoning him. "I want you to have this with you always, so I am writing it out. This is from Psalm 139: 'If I say, surely the darkness shall overwhelm me, and the light about me shall be night; even the darkness hideth not from thee, but the light shineth as the day: the darkness and the light are both alike to thee. For thou didst form my inward parts: thou didst cover me in my mother's womb. I will give thanks unto thee; for I am fearfully and wonderfully made: wonderful are thy works; and that my soul knoweth right well. My frame was not hidden from thee, when I was made in secret, and curiously wrought in the lowest parts of the earth. Thine eyes did see mine unformed substance; and in thy book they were written, even the days that were ordained for me, when as yet there was none of them. How precious also are thy thoughts unto me, O God! How great is the sum of them! If I should count them, they are more in number than the sand: when I awake, I am still with thee.'

"These words are just as though they were written for my baby and the thousands of other babies waiting to be born. I checked in another girl's Bible and hers says, "Thine eyes did see my substance, yet being imperfect; and in thy book all my members were written, which in continuance were fashioned, when as yet there was none of them." God *does* know our babies intimately. He is designing them, and He even knows beforehand what they will turn out to be. Don't you see, Daddy, that if God is knowing them before birth and knowing what their lives will be like, no man has the right to interfere with what He is doing? But, Dad, God must have told the Psalmist that Evil would try to destroy babies in the womb, because the very next verse goes on, 'Surely thou wilt slay the wicked, O God: depart from me therefore, ye bloodthirsty men.' The idea of continuance is important too. If life is begun with the capacity to continue to full growth, then interrupting that life at any point is equally heinous—one month along or nine months or forty years is a meaningless distinction. If life would have matured without intervention, then the artificial interruption of that continuum at *any* time is murder. Why all this fuss about *when*, Dad? I don't see any difference.

"But that's not the only place in the Bible that I've found God knowing us as persons long before we are born. God apparently creates us in His mind from the beginning of time. Paul points this out in Ephesians: '... he chose us in him before the foundation of the world, that we should be holy and without blemish before him in love' (1:4), and he re-emphasizes his point in 2:10, 'For we are his workmanship, created in Christ Jesus for good works, which God afore prepared that we should walk in them.' His foreknowledge of our lives and choices does not negate our free choices, of course, since He is God He knows all things and is not limited by our ideas of time and sequence.

"The gift of prophecy given to God's people clearly demonstrates that God conceives His human creations from an eternal stance, eons, centuries, generations before they are biologically conceived by man in woman. Consider His promise to Abraham: 'Look now toward heaven, and number the stars, if thou be able to number them: and he said unto him, So shall thy seed be' (Gen. 15:5). Or remember His covenant with David: 'And thy house and thy kingdom shall be made sure for ever before thee: thy throne shall be established for ever' (2 Sam. 7:16). Or think on His promises to the women in the Scriptures who desired children, the hospitable and wealthy wife of Shunem who had no son until Elisha spoke the Word of the Lord to her promising a son within a year's time; Hannah, who had no child until God promised through Eli the priest to grant the desire for which she so earnestly prayed; or Elizabeth, old and barren until God spoke to her husband the promise of a son, John, who would have many specifically described characteristics and who would have a set mission.

"Jeremiah was known to God before his conception: 'Now the word of Jehovah came unto me, saying, Before I formed thee in the belly I knew thee, and before thou camest forth out of the womb I sanctified thee' (Jer. 1:4-5). And Isaiah's son was planned by the Lord before conception and used as a sign. He was even *named* by the Lord before his conception (Isaiah 8). The relationship of Jacob and his twin brother Esau was foretold while they were yet struggling together in the womb. Later Jacob, in prophecy, was able to accurately foretell the destiny of the offspring of each of his twelve sons. Truly God knows us before our birth and before our physical conception. To be known and loved by God is to exist.

"You can see why I'm so excited over these Scriptures, Daddy, and why I want you to think about them. Who knows what God has planned for my baby or the babies of the poor women the government wants to help. I'm looking for more in my Bible. Thank you again for giving it to me. You'll be hearing from me! I love you."

The Twenty-eighth Week—Sorrow

I look like a wrinkled, little old man. Apparently my skin has been growing more rapidly than my underlying connective tissue. But I am starting to fatten up, and soon the rest of me should have caught up with my skin. I have my eyebrows and eyelashes now, and my face looks like a presentable infant. My brain probably has its full complement of brain cells; the cells will continue to increase in size until I am a year and a half old. The pupillary membranes are disappearing from my eyes. I am growing so fast that Mother can't zip her jeans *at all*. She has gotten some maternity clothes from the counselling center where the Nurse took Mother that first day of my reprieve.

Some hard things are happening to Mother now that everyone knows that she is expecting me by looking at her. A lot of the students snicker or laugh, and others just look away with embarrassment. She has been called in to talk with the Dean of Women who finally agreed that she could finish out the term although it was "highly irregular." Surprisingly, some of the meanest remarks are coming from the girls who Mother knows have had abortions themselves.

Two happenings hurt Mother the most. Roger, the Christian fellow who had been giving Mother a ride to church, called to tell her that he wouldn't be able to pick her up anymore. He said that he was going to have to get there real early to usher and wouldn't have time to come by for her, but Mother knew in her heart that he was ashamed to be seen coming in with her. She cried herself to sleep over this betrayal that night, because she thought her Christian friends would be different. Then the Holy Spirit taught her that her fellow believers were often weak and imperfect, even as she was, and that she needed to love and forgive Roger anyway.

The other hurt was much more deep and pervasive. It came in a cheerful and brave letter from Mother's mother. In part the letter read: "Of course, I respect your decision and we will stand with you through the consequences. I've given quite a bit of thought to the matter and have decided that it would be the least difficult and the most comfortable for you to go to your Aunt Peggy's when the school term is over. I've already talked with her, and she says that she and Uncle Al will welcome you into their home. It's far enough away from everywhere that you needn't worry about talk filtering back here. Joanie and I haven't said a word to anyone, so your secret is safe with us. I will come out to Peggy and Al's when your time comes so that I can be with you. Peggy knows a good O.B. there and thinks that two months will be plenty of time for you to make whatever plans you wish (in regard to the baby). We've already mentioned to some folks here that you may be working at one of the National Parks this summer on kind of a pre-naturalist internship. So study up hard on your flora and fauna facts! Joanie's prom dress is stunning—deep blue with lace inserts. She went with Johnny Baker and they . . . " Mother dropped the letter because she couldn't see the pages to read any more. She had planned to be at home . . . to be in her own room . . . to go to St. Joseph's Hospital. She had prayed that God would allow her to be a positive witness to His forgiveness and His redemptive love. Now it appeared that her mother didn't want her there—that her time of witness was to become a time of deception.

After awhile, the Holy Spirit, called the Comforter, broke through her tears. "Blessed are they that have been persecuted for righteousness' sake: for theirs is the kingdom of heaven." Where had she read that? Well, she was reaping the result of her own sin, not her righteousness. "Don't you have the righteousness of Christ now?" "Yes." "Are you not bearing this child to life now for my sake?" "Yes." "Blessed are they that have been persecuted for righteousness' sake." Mother sat up and began thumbing through her Bible. Her eye rested on Colossians 1:24 where Paul writes: "Now I rejoice in my sufferings for your sake, and fill up on my part that which is lacking of the afflictions of Christ in my flesh for his body's sake, which is the church; whereof I was made a minister, according to the dispensation of God . . . to make known . . . the riches of the glory of this mystery among the Gentiles, which is Christ in you, the hope of glory . . . that we may present every man perfect in Christ; whereunto I labor also, striving according to his working, which worketh in me mightily." Mother closed her eyes. She knew what St. Paul meant when he wrote those words. God was letting her do the same, in a different way. Christ was with her, in her, and her suffering on behalf of His body, the church, would allow her to present me to God. And then that still, small voice that was not audible reminded her, "Don't forget. My own Mother knew the pain of being an unwed mother for a time, even though she was a virgin. Your suffering can be a holy participation in my plan of salvation for your little one."

Mother fell asleep praying, "Jesus, help me to love my mother, just the way she is."

The Twenty-ninth Week—Daddy

The thing that Mother feared the worst has happened. My daddy found out. Some fellows from the University were visiting on Mother's campus, and when they went back they told him. He phoned Mother right away.

"Jill?"

Mother knew his voice, and I got a shot of adrenalin, slightly delayed. "Hello, Ben."

"Is it true that you're ... that you're ... "

"Yes, Ben. It's true."

"Why didn't you call me?"

"What for?"

"What do you mean, 'What for'?"

"We agreed not to see each other again."

"Yes, but this is different. I could have helped you to do something. I mean, I'm involved too, you know. I feel rotten that you didn't call me right away. Look, we've got to talk about this. I'm coming over tomorrow."

"I ... I don't want you to see me like this."

"C'mon, Jill. Don't be dumb. This is important. I'm coming tomorrow at 3:30. You be ready, for a change, okay?"

"I've got a lab until 4:30."

"I'll be there at quarter 'til five."

"Well, okay." Mother hung up the phone in a state of near panic. All the old emotions surrounding my daddy were bubbling up inside her. She started to pray, "Jesus, help me ... "

Mother's heart jumps when she sees Daddy standing in the dorm reception room. He is dark and slim and has a stylish haircut that emphasizes his heavy eyebrows.

"Hello, Ben. Did you get into law school for the fall?"

"Yes. Hello, Bitch." Mother cringes at the name even though she knows it's a term of affection from him.

"Did Daddy write you a good recommendation?"

"He must have. I got in. Where do you want to go? Are you hungry?" He shoots a quick glance toward Mother's stomach, and she can feel a blush rising. Mother starts to pray again.

"Let's just go for a ride and talk." They spend some time talking about mutual friends, their classes, and other inconsequential subjects.

Finally he swears and asks, "Jill, why are you doing this?"

"That's why."

"What do you mean?"

"I mean I'm doing it for God's sake. I know He wants the baby to live."

"How do you know that?"

"He's showed me, and I've become a Christian."

"What do you mean you've *become* a Christian? You always were. Are you getting religious on me or something?"

"No, Ben. But a person has to *decide* to live for God. It's not automatic. I've decided to make Jesus the Lord of my life." Mother is blushing again.

Daddy doesn't answer for a long time. He is looking directly into Mother's eyes. "I think you really have," he says finally. "Look, do you want to get married?"

"Shotgun weddings are passé."

"I'm not fooling around. If you're going to go through with this, we can't let the kid be a bastard.

If it doesn't work out we can get divorced later on."

"That would be just great," says Mother bitterly; "then who would take care of him?" She is immediately sorry for her words. "I'm sorry, Ben. I'm really touched that you are willing to get married. We . . . it just wouldn't work."

"Why not, Jill? We can get it together again like before. What about the baby? We've got to think about him."

"He's probably a her. I *am* thinking about the baby. I'm planning to give the baby up for adoption to a Christian family."

"Wait a minute . . . he's half mine . . . he's half Jewish."

"How come so proprietary all of a sudden? . . . Oh, Ben, I'm sorry again. I don't know what's the matter with me." Mother is being sorely tempted. She sees the curve of his arm at the steering wheel under his knit shirt, the determined look that comes over his face, the intelligence in his eyes—all of the attributes that made her love him in the first place. For a moment she lets her mind dwell on the picture that leaps to her mind—a cozy apartment, a ring on her finger, Ben next to her every night, Ben with her in the labor room holding her hand . . . "Ben, that's no way to start a marriage. I know now that I must wait until God chooses a husband for me and gives me a home—if He does. It wouldn't be right to get married unless it were a lifetime commitment. I can't ask that from you, and I couldn't give it to you right now. We're just not ready. We weren't ready before, and this certainly doesn't make us any more ready."

"I might grow up a whole lot when I'm a father."

"It's not your *fault*, Ben. And God is making it turn out for good, because now I love Him. You'll see."

"How about me? Do you still love me?"

"Ben—what a question . . . not like before. I love you now as a person Jesus loves and died for."

"What is *that* supposed to mean?"

Gently, gently, Mother is telling him about the real presence of God in her spirit, about the change in her mind-set, about the joy He is giving her in the midst of her trouble, about the love she is feeling for their unborn child—a sacrificial love that would give up anything for the baby's eternal welfare, even give up the baby himself. My daddy is listening quietly.

The Thirtieth Week—
The Spirit of the Age

Mother is writing to the Lawgiver again. "Dear Daddy: This is finals week and I should be studying but I just have to share some more of what I've been discovering in the Bible, because I want you to really think about it. The whole message of the Bible about children is that they are a tremendous blessing from the Lord—perhaps His best earthly blessing. Nowhere is a child considered less than God's marvelous gift for a man or a woman. Why is our culture turning away from this knowledge, Dad? My generation often has a soured and cynical view of children as a troublesome nuisance—the exact reverse of the truth. Is it that we have devalued our own lives so much, demeaned ourselves in our own eyes, denied the image of God in us to such an extent that we cannot value the human life we conceive? Why have we allowed ourselves to be so deceived?

" 'Lo, children are a heritage of Jehovah; and the fruit of the womb is his reward. As arrows in the hand of a mighty man, so are the children of youth. Happy is the man that hath his quiver full of them,' says Psalm 127:3-5. And 'Blessed is every one that feareth Jehovah, that walketh in his ways. For thou shalt eat the labor of thy hands: happy shalt thou be, and it shall be well with thee. Thy wife shall be as a fruitful vine, in the innermost parts of thy house; thy children like olive plants, round about thy table. Behold, thus shall the man be blessed that feareth Jehovah' (Ps. 128:1-4). These verses are directed toward the fathers, but here's one for us women, 'He maketh the barren woman to keep house, and to be a joyful mother of children' (Ps. 113:9). Someday, I pray, God will make that true for me.

"But while affirming the satisfaction and blessing of children, God makes it clear that the opposite, the lack of children or their death by miscarriage or later, is a sadness and a curse. When Abimelech unknowingly took Sarah, another man's wife, into his household, God caused all the wombs in his house to be barren until Abraham interceded with God for him and God restored their fertility (Gen. 20). Hosea says that part of the terrible punishment for corruption is that 'their glory shall fly away like a bird: there shall be no birth, and none with child, and no conception.' Do you see how Hosea lists two stages of pregnancy plus infertility? Obviously any one of the categories would have made his point, But he shows us that as a punishment for sin to the nation some will not be able to conceive, some will lose babies during early pregnancy ('none with child'), and others will lose babies just before birth. Hosea further implies that the 'miscarrying womb and dry breasts' are a sign of the Lord's casting away of His people. The Scriptures always view the loss of a baby as a horrendous sorrow. There is never even a hint that one would deliberately choose this evil and abort herself.

"Jesus predicted on His way to the cross that the days were coming when women would say, 'Blessed are the barren, and the wombs that never bare, and the breasts that never gave suck. Then shall they begin to say to the mountains, Fall on us, and to the hills, Cover us. For if they do these things in the green tree, what shall be done in the dry?' Perhaps the negative attitude we now see in regard to children is predictive that the end time is near. We are estranged from the blessing of fruitfulness from the Lord, and we don't even know what we are denying ourselves.

"The overall message of the Scriptures is the message of our Heavenly Father creating us, loving us, pitying us in our sin, chastising us as wayward children when we need it, redeeming us through Christ, guiding us, and caring for us tenderly. The spirit of parental love is so pervasive that nowhere does the Scripture even suggest the relationship of parent to child should be anything but a relationship like the Loving Creator-Parent to creature-child. *The Scriptures do not specifically condemn abortion by name because it is unthinkable.* The idea is totally opposed to God's Spirit of Fatherly Love that formed the universe and its inhabitants. Only the godless heathen sacrifice their sons and daughters, and that is because in their ignorance they are appeasing their wrathful gods with the most precious thing they have.

"When the spirit of the age begins to deny life, to hate children, to kill babies, then we must know for sure that the spirit at work is completely evil, opposed to the very nature of God as Father. Such a spirit of Evil is trying to destroy our nation, and every evidence is that unless we repent and change our hearts and our law, we *will* be devastated by Evil.

"Until I came to know my Father through Jesus, I could not see what spirit was behind the push to abort my child. I did not know that Evil was at work to deceive me and lead me to murder and to deny creation. As soon as the Holy Spirit entered me, I was enlightened, and I was able to have parental love like God's. Immediately the thought of killing a child, any child, was abhorrent to me. Dad, we can talk endlessly about morality, but until the Holy Spirit comes to open our eyes, we cannot see

Evil at work in us or in others. We keep trying to have good ethics without the Power that makes ethical life possible, even understandable. Men and women will never know that abortion is completely and always evil until they have received the Spirit of Life from the Father. Only when God gives me spiritual life do I recognize death at work. When I know my Father through Jesus, then I am freed to unmask the anti-life spirit. More on this later. Love, Jill."

The Thirty-first Week—Apology

Even though she is really pressed for time during this week of her final exams, Mother has discovered how essential daily Bible reading and prayer are to her well-being. "Heavenly Father, I give myself once more to you today to do Your will..." she begins to pray. Today she is reading in Matthew 5, "If therefore thou art offering thy gift at the altar, and there rememberest that thy brother hath aught against thee, leave there thy gift before the altar, and go thy way, first be reconciled to thy brother, and then come and offer thy gift." Then begins one of those internal conversations with the Holy Spirit that only the Christian understands. God starts in His inaudible voice, *"The Social Worker has something against you. You left her very rudely and without explanation in a way that could have caused her professional embarrassment. Even though she was very wrong, she was trying to help you."* "But, Lord, You know what she is better than I do!" *"She is someone I created and for whom redemption has been paid. I love her."* "What could I do about her now?" *"Go and ask her to forgive you for your rude behavior."* "She'll think I'm crazy, and it won't do any good. I'll be real nice to all social workers in the future." *"It is better to obey than to sacrifice."* "All right. I'll do it, but You're responsible if she throws me right out of her office.... Please help me with whatever You want me to say—and give me Your love for her, because I have none of my own."

Mother decides it would be better to go to the

mental health center without an appointment. Perhaps the Social Worker will be out or too busy to see her. But, as God would have it, the Social Worker is standing at the reception desk when Mother comes in. She takes Mother and me in with a glance and quickly puts on her professional stance.

"Hello, Jill. How are you doing?" She doesn't seem upset to see Mother. Maybe Mother just imagined that God told her to do this embarrassing thing.

"I'd like to talk with you if you have a few minutes free," says Mother.

"Certainly. Please come into my office. Do you want a Coke?"

"No, thank you," says Mother.

After they are seated in the office, Mother begins to feel very foolish indeed. "I . . . uh . . . I . . . uh . . . came to apologize for my behavior last time. I was rude to leave the way I did."

"Your apology is accepted. I understand why you were in an upset state. Are you ready now to talk things over again?"

"Uh . . . no. I just came to say I'm sorry. You see, I've become a Christian, and I needed to ask your forgiveness. There's nothing else to talk over. I've decided to choose life for my baby instead of death and to give him up for adoption to a Christian family."

"You've thought this through carefully and are aware of the problems this might cause you?" The Social Worker is looking uncomfortable.

"Yes, I have." Suddenly Mother is aware that she is feeling tremendous compassion for the Social Worker. She must know neither the Fatherhood of God nor the fatherhood of a good human father, or else she would not hate men as she does. "God will keep me through this time, and He is providing for my every need. He loves us as a father loves his children, you know." Whoops—that sounds like the wrong thing to say.

The Social Worker smiles and stands up to indicate that the impromptu interview is over. "Thanks for coming by," she says. "I wish you the best."

Mother leaves perplexed. Why had God told her to come? There was no perceptible change in the Social Worker. Mother's hope for a chance to witness to her new life in Christ was squelched. The whole interview seems a waste of time except for the feeling of relief that Mother has from obeying God. Mother will never know that she carried a very clear message from the Holy Spirit to the Social Worker, "If you hear my voice today, do not be stubborn, as your ancestors were when they rebelled against me. Return to me while there is yet time, for my spirit will not always strive with you." Mother was only one of four that God had sent to the Social Worker within a few days with the same hidden message.

The Social Worker picks up the phone and dials an outside line. "I'm not ready to come with you yet tonight. I need more time to think about it."

The Thirty-second Week—Transition

This is moving week for Mother and me. I don't know how Mother accumulated so much stuff. She is packing most of it away in boxes that will be stored here at college for her until next fall. She feels that she definitely wants to come back here so that she can show with her life how Jesus really redeems, changes, and vitalizes a person.

Meanwhile, I have considerable progress of my own to report. I am a red-skin right now, and covered with *vernix caseosa*, a cheesy-looking, greasy substance that is made up of my sloughed-off skin cells and sebaceous secretion. This goop protects my skin from irritation by the amniotic fluid around me. My eyelids are no longer fused shut. My lanugo hair all over is beginning to disappear, but the hair on my head is growing longer and thicker. *If* I am a boy (and I won't tell) my left testicle has begun its descent into the scrotum. My intestines have some dark green stuff in them called meconium which is a mixture of bile, mucus, and epithelial cells. I have fattened up considerably under my skin so that I don't look wrinkled anymore. In fact, I would say I have well-rounded contours.

Personality-wise, I have a little bit of scaredy-cat in me, because when I hear a loud sound my heart will begin to beat faster. I also get the hiccups sometimes. My sucking instinct is getting stronger. I will turn my head toward a stimulus and reach out my lips. If an electroencephalogram (a picture of my brain wave activity) were done next week, it would show that I have three definite kinds of brain activity which are recognizable patterns; these three patterns are like the adult patterns of sleep, wakefulness, and dreaming sleep (rapid eye movement sleep). The things I dream about are things of the spirit—unutterable—but God is teaching me then. If I were to be born prematurely now, I definitely could live. I weigh over 1500 grams! That's almost three and a half pounds. From now on my tissues will be built up but no new tissue will develop.

A very touching thing happened. The girls on Mother's dorm floor gave her a shower. It couldn't be a regular baby shower for me, because they all know that I am going to be someone else's baby, and that other mother will want to plan a layette for me. But Mother's friends wanted Mother to have some receiving blankets, a pretty crib blanket, some tiny booties, and a few pastel gowns to take to the hospital so that whoever took me home with them would know that I was dearly loved. They understand that Mother is sacrificing for me, and their hearts have been strangely moved by the Life of Jesus in Mother that is helping her to make way for a secure life for me. Some have said to her, "I couldn't do it, Jill—all the ridicule and then the physical pain you'll have to go through." Mother answers that she couldn't either without Jesus. Many of the girls have given very serious thought to the question of abortion because of Mother's example. In fact, a few of them have started a small referral service on campus called simply Alternatives. They have gotten some pro-life materials and have succeeded in placing them in the campus clinic and in the girls' restrooms around campus.

All of the good-byes and best wishes and admonitions to write *immediately* to tell if I'm a boy or a girl and anything that Mother finds out about my new family make Mother feel very happy. But she sets out for the flight to Aunt Peggy's house with some trepidation. Aunt Peggy had sent Mother a warm letter telling her that they love her and are looking forward to two whole months of her company. She is to have the guest room and can use Buddy's car because he is in Mexico for the summer on a missionary project. Missionary project? Her cousin Buddy? She cannot imagine Buddy as any kind of missionary.

Aunt Peggy is her father's sister. The only lasting impression of Aunt Peggy and Uncle Al that she carries from her childhood is how much they loved each other. Funny how an emotional climate in a home makes a lasting impression. They didn't seem to fight like her mom and dad. She hasn't seen them for four years. Her cousin Sally was about twelve then and had braces on her teeth, and Buddy was a goofy guy of fifteen. Mother's mom and dad had visited since then, and now her dad sees them fairly often when in that part of the country on business.

Both Aunt Peggy and Uncle Al are at the landing gate. They give us a warm hug. As they talk with Mother on the way to the baggage area and during the long ride in the car, Mother begins to relax. How wonderful it seems that Aunt Peggy and Uncle Al love one another more now than ever.

The Thirty-third Week—The Plan

Today Aunt Peggy and Mother went to the adoption agency that "just happens" to be in this town. I have a definite feeling that God is very actively arranging my future according to His perfect plan for me. The social worker at the agency is a delightful woman who obviously loves babies (what a relief!). She quickly determines that Mother does not need financial assistance, medical help, a Christian foster home in which to live, or extra emotional support— these things are available for those mothers-to-be who need them. She is very careful to be sure that Mother has decided that adoption is the very best plan for me and encourages Mother to express any reservations she might have. Mother tells her that she has come to love me very much and that is why she wants to be sure that I go to a family that will rear me as a Christian child in a loving, solid home.

The social worker smiles, "That's what we want, too," she assures Mother, "if you decide to put your child in an adoptive home." The social worker says that Mother will have plenty of time before she signs a final release for me. A temporary foster home that just loves babies will care for me until Mother is absolutely sure she wants me to be with the Christian family. The foster family will give me their own pet name but my permanent family will never know what it was. My foster family will also keep a diary of my daily doings so that my new parents will be up to date when I first go home. I'm glad someone will keep up my journal! Mother will be able to see me after I'm born, if she wants to check me out.

I'd like to feel and smell and hear Mother from the outside, too.

Just a week with Aunt Peggy, Uncle Al, and Sally has crystallized Mother's mental picture of what a joyful Christian home can be—for, yes, her aunt and uncle and Sally are all Christians too. How did she miss that knowledge altogether when she was younger? They just seemed like a normal happy family and she had never asked herself *why* they were happy. Mother is beginning to understand why the Lord did not allow her to return home this summer. He is so good, and so infinitely much wiser than she. With a jolt Mother realized that her own father had known how she would feel as a new Christian because he knew his own Christian sister well. That's why he brought the study Bible. And, perhaps, her mom knew that Aunt Peggy has a strength to share with Mother that her own mom does not have—perhaps mom really *does* want her at home but doesn't feel she could help as much as Aunt Peggy can during this difficult time.

The social worker is asking Mother a lot of questions about herself, her family, my daddy, and his family. She also is writing down my daddy's address because he needs to consent in writing to my release. She even asks for a complete description of what Daddy looks like! She will talk again with Mother in a couple of weeks. She promises Mother that she will tell her about my new family, but not enough to identify them. She writes down the name of Mother's new physician and knows which hospital Mother will be at when she brings me to birth and the approximate date. The social worker says she will be there herself on the occasion of my nativity if she possibly can.

The social worker tells Mother that many Christian couples are praying for a baby to love and that she is sure that God has picked out my future family with great care, if indeed He continues to lead Mother to give me for adoption. She assures Mother that although the agency makes a careful registry of all the pertinent data from the natural parents and the prospective adoptive parents in order to do a good matching, the task is approached with much prayer, and she feels that God does the final matching, for "God setteth the solitary in families" (Ps. 68:6).

Aunt Peggy is taking Mother out to lunch at a nice restaurant to celebrate. Yes, to celebrate God's redeeming Love. God is so good, and we can trust Him totally with our lives. Aunt Peggy makes Mother order milk for me instead of iced tea. Mother assures her that she has been very careful about my proper nutrition all along. Mother feels free enough now to ask Aunt Peggy some questions about labor and childbirth and to mention what came as quite a shock and concern to her—Ben will have to sign release papers for me or else deny that I am his child. What if he won't?

The Thirty-fourth Week—Father

Uncle Al is such a cut-up I may come early if he doesn't quit making Mother laugh so hard at supper. After cleaning up the dishes with Sally, Mother decides to go to her room to write her father again instead of watching television. She has been thinking deeply about a father's role in the family for the past few days and talking about it with Aunt Peggy. "Daddy," she begins her letter, "thank you for being a real father to me and Joanie. I've been thinking so much about how important a father is to his family. Each of us is created to be an eternal child of the Heavenly Father. We live an earthly life from babyhood to old age that is specifically and personally designed to teach us to be the child that He desires. When we come to spiritual maturity and know brotherhood with our Lord Jesus Christ, we are, together with Him, forever children of the Heavenly Father. Jesus shows us how to be the sons and daughters of our Father.

"The Creator has set the people of earth in families that we might from our earliest natural moments begin to learn our ways as an eternal child. Our bodies and minds and lives are patterned into a family paradigm, or model, and our wills—the freely choosing part of us—are given a concrete insight into the intended eternal relationship of our Heavenly Father and us as obedient and loving children. Our wills may then choose the graceful entry into that eternal child-life with the Father or reject that eternity for the unknown non-family of self-will and un-love.

"The eternal spirit that God has breathed into each

living person is itself breathlessly awaiting the decision of the will in regard to accepting eternal life through Jesus. Will I to live, or not? The will *must* be accurately informed of the crucial reality and eternal consequences of its choice. The will receives information by the direct intuition of the Spirit, surely, but also through the mind via the person's own life experiences and observations. The will must decide whether or not his own eternal soul created by the Father for His own family will be in that family forever. The choice is between a son-life with God or separation from Him. The mind forms its opinion about what a father-child union (or disunion) is like through experience. Hopefully that opinion is that a father gives peace, structure, purpose, order, support, guidance, freedom to grow, encouragement, appreciation, discipline, and total love to his child. You did that for me, Daddy. When I hear the word "father" I experience again all of those good things. That is why the idea of an eternal child life with the Heavenly Father who is perfectly all of those good qualities and infinitely more is a true and appealing idea to me. My will was inclined to choose life when the Holy Spirit called me to an eternal life with the Father. I love the idea of father because I love you.

"But for some people the will has no good experience or observation of a father. Or the will may have an ugly, hateful, fearful unpredictable idea of a father and might choose death as preferable. Clearly our families on earth are exceedingly more than a societal convention. They are a vital communication link that allows the mind to form an idea of father that will help the will to choose Father and eternal life when the Holy Spirit speaks. The way to the Father is openly shown by His Son Jesus, our Savior, who himself has paid the price of His righteous blood for our adoption as sons. Daddy, it would be so sad if even one soul refused to submit to the mastery of Christ and the Fatherhood of God because of a faulty mental model of father and child.

"I know that healthy human personality is formed almost exclusively in the nurture of an intact family; there is no substitute for a family. God's concern and compassion for the fatherless is everywhere in the Scriptures, and their welfare is to be urgent upon the heart of the Christian. Sometimes a child becomes fatherless through death or divorce at an early period in his life. I think in that circumstance the Christian mother would need to speak frequently of the Heavenly Father and His care and find other Christian men who will take a fatherly interest in the child. Jesus himself will come to complete the home when He is asked.

"But what I'm getting around to, Daddy (maybe I'm trying to convince myself!), is that as much as I would like to be a mother right now to my baby, a good father is absolutely essential for his mental and spiritual well-being. Yes, God will fill in the psychological gaps when necessary. But, in my case, to choose to handicap my baby by keeping him myself without a father would be very, very selfish. I am committed to giving him/her up for adoption to a real family. Somehow it just helps to write out these thoughts on paper.

"So I just want to say thanks, Dad, for being a real father. I pray that my baby will have a father like you. I love you."

The Thirty-fifth Week—Negotiation

Mother has decided to write to my daddy before he is notified by the adoption agency and is asked to relinquish his rights to me. After some false starts she stops to pray and then writes: "Dear Benji: When we talked before you'll remember I told you of my plans to give our baby up for adoption. I have made the initial arrangements with a marvelous agency here where my aunt and uncle live. I wanted to explain to you why I have gone ahead with a Christian agency. They choose their adoptive parents with a careful eye for a spiritual commitment to God and to one another. As you know, the stress on families these days is horrendous, and family stability is essential for a healthy personality to grow. I don't think a family can stay together without the spiritual dimension in these pressured times.

"Many people simply do not know how to be godly parents—parents who will reflect God's attributes of law, love, and mercy to little persons. Possibly they have not learned themselves to be a child before God, and so they cannot teach their offspring to be a child before Him. Maybe their own parents were poor models of fatherliness and motherliness. But the Heavenly Father looks for those who desire to do His will and is right there to help when He is called upon. If the agency selects an inexperienced couple seeking His way, He can first teach them the meaning of childhood and then He can make them into fitting images of Himself and models for the child. Of course, many of the couples will already be mature Christians. Either way, our child has a good chance for a stable homelife.

"But, Ben, I fear that a couple without a spiritual commitment might succumb to the evil anti-child spirit that is gripping our nation, even though at first they sincerely desire to adopt a child. Without the Spirit of God they could not resist the influence of this invading spirit. As our society increasingly devalues our own personhood by denying the eternal spirit-person within our body and soul (the mind, emotion, and will matrix), new persons also lose their value to us. If we are but a complex product of chemistry doomed to a short, self-actuating, organic life, we are expendable. Babies, children, the handicapped, the infirm, the aged are especially expendable since they do not serve our fleshly desires, but rather use up the time and resources better spent on orgiastic pleasure. This kind of godless reasoning is rampant today, especially among the sophisticates.

"The anti-child spirit in our midst convinces many young couples to choose to be 'child-free' so that they might pursue their own worldly goals exclusively and have no need to share in the formation of new life. Many couples simply postpone children until their materialistic appetites are sated; that satiation may never come. World over-population is cited as a primary motive for non-childrearing, yet few or none so concerned contribute time, money, or selves to the rearing of unparented children already here. The anti-child spirit has succeeded in polluting our land with the blood of millions of aborted children in the name of population control, mental health, women's rights, or 'reproductive freedom.'

"The anti-child spirit has shunted millions of small persons into impersonal day care centers when their hearts and emerging personalities desperately need the consistency of one mother and a warm, orderly environment. The anti-child spirit allows *any* other selfish need to take precedence over the emotional needs of children or teens. The driving force behind the anti-child spirit desires to rob the Heavenly Father of His created children, either by murdering them outright or by starving them emotionally so that as psychological cripples they cannot grasp the glory of belonging to the Father.

"That's why we want a couple who hold God's views on the value of personhood to be parents for our baby. Most of the couples who seek to adopt a baby through any agency are probably going to be loving parents, because it shows a lot of motivation to wait that long for a child, but, Ben, I want to be *sure* that our baby has God-fearing parents. We are united on this value, I believe, Ben. If our situation were reversed, I would allow our child to go to a God-fearing Jewish couple. We must not quibble theologically when we agree on life *versus* death.

"I am concerned for you personally too. The Heavenly Father will not be thwarted in His loving purpose of calling all Israel to Him. Please, please look in the Scriptures for the prophecies about the Messiah. He is the One who gives the Power to create families that are life-long and loving. The best of sincere intent to make a good family is not enough without the spiritual power that comes from God. I'm sure that someday God will want to make a patriarch out of you, Ben! But I'm sure that God's will now is to place our baby in a godly family that will cherish him. Love . . ."

The Thirty-sixth Week—
Bible Study

My stay here with Mother has focused the attention of Aunt Peggy, Uncle Al, Sally, and some of their Christian friends on the issue of what they might be doing to affirm God's position on the sanctity of life. Uncle Al is horrified to discover that his own Christian denomination has adopted in convention an anti-life platform with the grievously mistaken rationale that the law must prevent discrimination against the poor in this area and must provide freedom of choice, and that morality cannot be legislated. "The poor as well as the rich must be allowed to murder? The poor must have unlimited freedom to choose Evil and death and guilt at government expense and with the sanction of the government? If the law does not protect life, why *have* any law?" fumes Uncle Al.

At first he is intensely angry at his denominational leaders and convention delegates for being so easily deceived by glib phrases and for not really thinking through the issue of abortion from a Biblical perspective. But then he is overcome by remorse when he realizes that he has not searched the Scriptures either. Perhaps he might be as easily deceived if he were not attending to the Holy Spirit within him. Al knows that although the Holy Spirit is always present in him to teach him, sometimes he doesn't stop to listen—he is a very busy and successful man. He may never ask the questions.

Uncle Al suggests that he, Peggy, Sally, and

Mother join in a thorough search of God's Word. He plans to begin speaking to his brothers and sisters in Christ about this great evil in our land that most of us simply ignore. Mother is thrilled that they will join her in her Bible study; she needs more to tell her father, the Lawgiver. They settle in around the oak table after dinner.

Uncle Al likes to use the Revised Standard Version of the Bible. "Here are some key verses that make the choice between life and death very clear," begins Al. "This is God speaking in Deuteronomy 30:15-20. 'See, I have set before you this day life and good, death and evil. If you obey the commandments of the Lord your God, by walking in his ways, and by keeping his commandments and his statutes and his ordinances, then you shall live and multiply, and the Lord your God will bless you in the land. . . . I call heaven and earth to witness against you this day, that I have set before you life and death, blessing and curse; therefore choose life, that you and your descendants may live, loving the Lord your God, obeying his voice, and cleaving to him. . . .' "

"Dad," asks Sally, "does that mean that when a country is purposely killing off its descendants that God's blessing has left?"

"The country is at least on its way to losing God's blessing, Sally. We may still have the option of choosing life. I hope so." Later on in Deuteronomy the curses are being read aloud to the people (27:25). One of them is 'Cursed be he who takes a bribe to slay an innocent person.' "

"Here's a verse like that in Exodus, too," adds Anut Peggy. " 'Keep far from a false charge, and do not slay the innocent and righteous, for I will not acquit the wicked.' Wait . . . it goes on, 'And you shall take no bribe, for a bribe blinds the officials, and subverts the cause of those who are in the right.' I think a lot of us are being bribed by the promise of fewer kids on welfare, fewer of the 'undesirable' element of society being born, fewer maternity cases to be funded by government funds, fewer mouths to eat up the produce of the land, and so on."

"How could we do anything about it?" asks Sally.

"I think that we can count on God to give us the strength to do whatever we must," Mother answers. "Let me show you what I found in two places in Proverbs. May I use that Bible? First, 24:10-12, 'If you faint in the day of adversity, your strength is small. Rescue those who are being taken away to death, hold back those who are stumbling to the slaughter. If you say, "Behold, we did not know this," does not he who weighs the heart perceive it? Does not he who keeps watch over your soul know it, and will he not requite man according to his work?' The other one, in chapter 30, verses 11 to 14, is really deep. This tells us that people who hate their own parents will tend to kill the children of the poor. 'There are those who curse their fathers and do not bless their mothers. There are those who are pure in their own eyes but are not cleansed of their filth. There are those—how lofty are their eyes, how high their eyelids lift! There are those whose teeth are swords, whose teeth are knives, to devour the poor from off the earth, the needy from among men.' " There is a stunned silence around the old oak table.

Finally, Uncle Al says, "Possibly all of those 'those's' do not refer to the same group of people. But it pretty well tells us how some supposedly religious people, or ethical people who don't know the forgiveness of Jesus, can plead as though they are for the rights of the poor while actually in their deepest hearts they are trying to kill them off through abortions."

"Wow," says Sally. "That makes me sick."

"I'm truly concerned for our church," says Uncle Al. "Jeremiah brought the scourging Word of the Lord to the church people when they were trusting their church structure for salvation while ignoring God's Law. He says in chapter 7:4-8, 'Do not trust in these deceptive words: "This is the temple of the Lord, the temple of the Lord, the temple of the Lord." For if you truly amend your ways and your doings, if you truly execute justice one with another, if you do not oppress the alien, the fatherless, or the widow, or shed innocent blood in this place, and if you do not go after other gods to your own hurt, then I will let you dwell in this place, in the land that I gave of old to your fathers forever. Behold, you trust in deceptive words to no avail. . . .' "

"Speaking of other gods," says Aunt Peggy, "did you know that one of our Supreme Court justices actually cited 'ancient religion' as a precedent for murdering babies in the womb?"

"No, I didn't know that," answers Uncle Al thoughtfully.

"I'm concerned for Daddy," says Mother. "He's right at the source of our lawmaking. Listen to what Isaiah says in chapter 10:1-4, 'Woe to those who decree iniquitous decrees, and the writers who keep writing oppression, to turn aside the needy from justice and to rob the poor of my people of their right, that widows may be their spoil, and that they may make the fatherless their prey! What will you do on the day of punishment, in the storm which will come from afar? To whom will you flee for help, and where will you leave your wealth? Nothing remains but to crouch among the prisoners or fall among the slain.' "

"Let's pray for your dad right now and for our other lawmakers," suggests Aunt Peggy, "that they may be true ministers of God for righteousness and protect the unborn."

After the prayer Uncle Al looks thoughtful again. "That reminds me of one more crucial passage," he says. "It's in Psalm 106; God is talking about His own people, Israel. 'They sacrificed their sons and daughters to the demons; they poured out innocent blood, the blood of their sons and daughters, whom they sacrificed to the idols of Canaan; and the land was polluted with blood . . . then the anger of the Lord was kindled against his people; and he abhorred his heritage; he gave them into the hand of the nations, so that those who hated them ruled over them. Their enemies oppressed them, and they were brought into subjection under their power.' "

"I sure hope that doesn't happen here," says Sally.

The Thirty-seventh Week—Covenant

We heard about my prospective parents today, Mother and I. He is an accountant and she is a school teacher who will not return to teaching in the fall if they get me. They live in a small town—not this one—and are active in their church. More important, they love Jesus. Both are in their late twenties, and they have been married for six years. The husband is dark and slender with heavy eyebrows. The wife is a small woman, pretty and vivacious. They have been waiting for a baby to love for a long time. In fact they have made up a nursery, a bright and sunny upstairs corner room in their home, but it's been empty for many months. They also have a big, shaggy dog.

Mother is feeling a pang of jealousy as she hears about their happy marriage. It is the desire of her heart to have a happy marriage, a home of her own, and children to rear for the Lord. But God reminds her of the promise in Psalm 37:4-5, "Delight thyself also in Jehovah; and he will give thee the desires of thy heart. Commit thy way unto Jehovah; trust also in him, and he will bring it to pass. And he will make thy righteousness to go forth as the light, and thy justice as the noonday. Rest in Jehovah, and wait patiently for him." She has told the Lord that she will be His handmaiden to bring me to life and has asked Him to prepare her to be someday a loving wife and the mother of her own Christian family. She knows in her heart that God has heard her prayer.

When we arrive home from the adoption agency,

there is a letter from my daddy, written with a black felt-tip pen on every other line of yellow lined paper. "Okay, Babe," it says in part, "I'll agree to whatever adoption agency you choose at this late point in the procedure. Let's hope he gets a better set of parents than we could be—at least right now. In living memory of you I'm going to a Jews for Jesus rally on the Island tonight with a guy from work. So you'd better pray for me!" Mother *is* praying for him.

Aunt Peggy is in the middle of a predicament. Her brother (my grandfather) called to say that he would be out for Mother's time of delivery. Aunt Peggy is supposed to phone him immediately at the first signs of my imminent arrival. He assumes that he will stay at Peggy and Al's house as he usually does. The problem is that my grandmother has been planning to come to their house too. Aunt Peggy is not going to choose between her brother and her sister-in-law, despite their estrangement. Neither does she want to permit a stressful situation to occur at the time Mother most needs calm and peaceful support. She can just imagine Mother's parents getting into one of their uproars if both came because of some false labor pains, and Mother might still be at home. Aunt Peggy and Uncle Al talk it over and pray about it. Then she writes a note to each of them.

"I have made reservations for both of you (separate rooms, of course) at the Ambassador which is not too far from the hospital. We'll give you Buddy's car to come back and forth to our house for dinners and for driving to the hospital. This is the best solution I could come up with to preserve the peace and serenity of your daughter. She is doing remarkably well. She needs all of our love and support at this time especially, and I know you don't want to cause her any anxiety. Please trust me that this is best. We love both of you very much and are looking forward to seeing you again." She seals the envelopes with a sigh.

Who knows what God might do at the Ambassador in response to prayer? Aunt Peggy is remembering the words from Malachi 2:14-16, ". . . the Lord was witness to the covenant between you and the wife of your youth, to whom you have been faithless, though she is your companion and your wife by covenant. Has he not made one and sustained for us the spirit of life? And what does he desire? Godly offspring. So take heed to yourselves, and let none be faithless to the wife of his youth. For I hate divorce, says the Lord the God of Israel, and covering one's garment with violence, says the Lord of hosts. So take heed to yourselves and do not be faithless."

The Thirty-eighth Week— Bloodbath

I've neglected my progress report in these last few exciting weeks. I'm nearly ready now. My skin is smooth; my fingernails have grown past the ends of my fingers and my tiny toenails are just at the ends of my toes. I'm quite plump, actually, and my legs have grown rapidly lately, but they won't be as long as my arms even by my birthday. All that lanugo hair on my body has disappeared. *If* I am a boy, both testes have descended into the scrotum. Probably all of my nerve cells have multiplied out, but they will continue to grow and specialize in function and organize themselves in layers in my brain. A lot of the cells don't know their special function yet, but my Father knows.

Right now I weigh almost seven pounds, and I am twenty inches long. My skull size is about thirteen inches around. My skull bones have soft spots between them that have not ossified; God has planned that my head can shift shape if necessary during my birth. My chest and my abdomen are about equal in size and are smaller around than my head. My sitting up height is about twelve or thirteen inches. But now I'm standing on my head, upside-down, waiting to be born. I am the subject of much interested speculation, and I'm getting eager to make my appearance. Mother has her suitcase packed and visits the doctor's office every week now.

Sally is causing some consternation at the dinner table tonight. "I talked with a girl at school today who actually had an abortion," she says. "I told her what we've been finding in the Bible."

"Wait a minute, Honey," says Uncle Al. "Did you also tell her about the forgiveness for *all* sin that is ours in Jesus Christ?"

"No, I didn't," says Sally, a bit shakily.

"Well, you need to talk to her immediately about God's forgiveness then, Honey. All of us sin in one way or another. If she has allowed her child to die it was a very grievous sin, but she is no worse off than any of us were before we came to the cross for forgiveness. Be *sure* to tell her that God loves her very much and has a special plan for her life."

"I will, Daddy," promises Sally.

"Knowing you are forgiven from a sin that really weighs on you is a fantastic relief," adds Mother. "Forgiveness changes a person's whole outlook on life. It makes you love God a whole lot, and it makes you want to quit sinning ever again. If she doesn't believe you, tell her I'll talk with her about it."

"Did you know that Psalm 51 was written by David in repentance for his sins of adultery and murder that caused the death of the little baby that was begotten by that adultery?" asks Aunt Peggy.

"No, I didn't!" says Mother, and she quickly goes to get a Bible to find the Psalm. "Oh, this is just great . . . Wow! . . . This is perfect . . . Yeah, man, that's just the way it is . . . Yes, tell her about this one, Sally!"

"Will you hurry up and read it out*loud*?" asks Sally, exasperated.

Her mother and father laugh. Mother reads, "Have mercy on me, O God, according to thy steadfast love; according to thy abundant mercy blot out my transgressions. Wash me thoroughly from my iniquity, and cleanse me from my sin! For I know my transgressions, and my sin is ever before me. Against thee, thee only, have I sinned, and done that which

is evil in thy sight, so that thou art justified in thy
sentence and blameless in thy judgment. Behold, I
was brought forth in iniquity, and in sin did my mother conceive me. Behold, thou desirest truth in the inward being; therefore teach me wisdom in my secret
heart. Purge me with hyssop, and I shall be clean;
wash me, and I shall be whiter than snow. Fill me
with joy and gladness; let the bones which thou hast
broken rejoice. Hide thy face from my sins, and blot
out all my iniquities. Create in me a clean heart, O
God, and put a new and right spirit within me. Cast
me not away from thy presence, and take not thy holy
spirit from me. Restore to me the joy of thy salvation,
and uphold me with a willing spirit. Then I will teach
transgressors thy ways, and sinners will return to
thee. Deliver me from bloodguiltiness, O God, thou
God of my salvation, and my tongue will sing aloud
of thy deliverance. O Lord, open thou my lips, and
my mouth shall show forth thy praise. For thou hast
no delight in sacrifice; were I to give a burnt offering,
thou wouldst not be pleased. The sacrifice acceptable
to God is a broken spirit; a broken and contrite heart,
O God, thou wilt not despise."

"What does 'purge me with hyssop' mean?" asks
Sally.

"At the time of the Jewish Passover in Egypt,
God instructed each Israelite family to take the blood
of their Passover lamb and to apply it with a hyssop
branch to the top and sides of their door. This would
make the sign of the cross in blood. God knew that
Jesus, the Lamb of God whose blood cleanses us
all from sin, would die on the cross. The blood of
the Passover lamb represented the blood of Christ,
and the Israelites were preserved from death that
night," Uncle Al explains. "When David writes 'purge
me with hyssop, and I shall be clean,' he is asking
God to wash him with the blood of the Eternal Lamb

of God, the blood of Jesus, for that is the only way we receive forgiveness of sin."

"What I really identify with is his joy from the Holy Spirit when he is forgiven, and his fantastic desire to praise and thank God," says Mother, with a catch in her voice. "And notice how he feels that he can teach other sinners about forgiveness, now that he is forgiven."

The Thirty-ninth Week—Manifesto

Mother has been preparing a special letter for her father for some weeks. Now it is time to send it. She has written to her mom too, of course, but notes to mom are more frequent, more newsy, more detailed, more everyday chronicles. Her mom will be arriving at the end of next week, unless summoned earlier. Joanie is staying at home with friends because she has a summer job. She spent some of her proceeds to send Mother a new nightgown with matching slippers for the hospital.

"Dear Daddy," the letter begins. "I've planned this letter for you to save and to read on the airplane when you are flying to this obscure place to be with me and your grandchild. I know how busy you are with matters of great importance to our government, and I'm so proud that God has put you in your place of responsibility. If you save this for the airplane flight, you'll be able to really concentrate and ponder these Bible words that I've found for you. Ready? Seat belt buckled?

"The first principle is that *all life comes exclusively from God and belongs to Him.* The Old Testament affirms this principle in many places, but for the sake of brevity I'll quote only one, Psalm 104:29-30, 'Thou hidest thy face, they [all living things] are troubled; thou takest away their breath, they die. Thou sendest forth thy Spirit, they are created. . . .' Saint Paul restates this principle in his speech to the Greeks in Athens (Acts 17:25) and adds that God also decides *how long* we live and *where* and that the express purpose of life is for man to have the opportunity to seek God and thus find eternal life: '. . . he himself giveth to all life, and breath, and all things; and he made of one every nation of men to dwell on all the face of the earth, having determined their appointed seasons, and the bounds of their habitation; that they should seek God, if haply they might feel after him and find him, though he is not far from each one of us: for in him we live, and move, and have our being. . . .' We must consider that to abort a baby is to deny him not only earthly life but eternal life. Abortion is the usurpation of God's exclusive prerogative of deciding life and death.

"The second principle is that *God knows us as unique persons while we are yet in the womb.* Not only does He make us in the womb, as we see in many Scriptures like Isaiah 44:24, 'Thus saith Jehovah, thy Redeemer, and he that formed thee from the womb: I am Jehovah, that maketh all things; that stretcheth forth the heavens alone; that spreadeth abroad the earth,' but also we have our created personalities in the womb. Consider Jacob, who, Hosea tells us in 12:3, 'in the womb . . . took his brother by the heel; and in his manhood he had power with God.' Saint Paul reminds us that God 'separated me even from my mother's womb, and called me through his grace, to reveal his Son in me . . .' (Gal. 1:15). Prenatal personality is shown even more clearly in the example of John the Baptist of whom it was said, 'He shall be filled with the Holy Spirit, even from his mother's womb.' His mother, Elizabeth, when six months pregnant, tells Mary, ' . . . behold, when the voice of thy salutation came into mine ears, the babe leaped in my womb for joy.'

"The third principle is that *God values all human life equally* (this ought to appeal to your egalitarian bias!). Job writes long, long ago, 'Did not he that made me in the womb make him [the servant of

Job]? And did not one fashion us in the womb?' And God desires that *every* man come to Him for salvation, ' . . . God our Saviour . . . would have all men to be saved, and come to the knowledge of the truth' (1 Tim. 2:3-4). Our Constitution provides us with the equal protection of the Law, not the equal opportunity to be helplessly murdered before birth.

"The fourth principle is that *God charges the government with the preservation of the children of the poor.* Psalm 72, for instance, describes the ruler who has God's righteousness and His judgments: 'He will judge thy people with righteousness, and thy poor with justice. . . . He will judge the poor of the people, he will save the children of the needy, and will break in pieces the oppressor. . . . For he will deliver the needy when he crieth, and the poor that hath no helper. He will have pity on the poor and needy, and the souls of the needy he will save. He will redeem their soul from oppression and violence; and precious will their blood be in his sight: and they shall live.'

"The fifth principle is that *God specifically defines an evil government as one that condemns innocent blood by law, and God will move to act against the nation that sheds the innocent blood of the poor* (or any innocent blood, for that matter). Psalm 94 lays it all out: 'Jehovah, how long shall the wicked, how long shall the wicked triumph? They prate, they speak arrogantly: all the workers of iniquity boast themselves. They break in pieces thy people, O Jehovah, and afflict thy heritage. They slay the widow and the sojourner, and murder the fatherless. And they say, "Jehovah will not see, neither will the God of Jacob consider." Consider, ye brutish among the people, and ye fools, when will ye be wise? He that planted the ear, shall he not hear? He that formed the eye, shall he not see? He that chastiseth the nations, shall not he correct, even he that teacheth man knowledge? Jehovah knoweth the thoughts of man, that they are vanity. Blessed is the man whom thou chastiseth, O Jehovah, and teachest out of thy law, that thou mayest give him rest from the days of adversity, until the pit be digged for the wicked. Who will rise up for me against the evil-doers? Who will stand up for me against the workers of iniquity? . . . Shall the throne of wickedness have fellowship with thee, which frameth mischief by statute? They gather themselves together against the soul of the righteous, and condemn innocent blood.' Notice especially the words 'break in pieces thy people' and 'afflict thy heritage' and 'murder the fatherless,' and notice the mention of God as the One who 'planted the ear' and 'formed the eye.' Don't these words make this Psalm searingly applicable to abortion?

"But God makes a promise in Psalm 9: 'For he that maketh inquisition for blood remembereth them; he forgetteth not the cry of the poor . . . The wicked shall be turned back unto [Hell], even all the nations that forget God. For the needy shall not always be forgotten, nor the expectation of the poor perish forever.'

"Daddy, I know from personal experience just a little of the psychological pain of carrying an unplanned child. Yet I know we must all reawaken as a nation to the reality of the utter sanctity of human life. Sacrifice and sorrow and inconvenience are part of what each of us must bear at some time in life that others might live. God *will* give the grace to go through any circumstance that He allows if we ask Him. Jesus said that 'a woman when she is in travail hath sorrow, because her hour is come: but when she is delivered of the child, she remembereth no more the anguish, for the joy that a man is born into the world' (John 16:21). I know that the other kind of sorrow, the kind that precedes labor, will be forgotten too in the splendor of that joy.''

The Fortieth Week—Quest

Today is my birthday. I am filled with a mixture of wild anticipation and undulating apprehension. What will the earth be like? She must be beautiful, for my Father has created her with great care and has imprinted her with visible reminders of His spiritual reality. But I know that Evil has not yet been removed from the earth, and I will have to overcome Evil during my lifetime by becoming one with the Victor who has overcome. God is telling me that my spirit will be in a sleep-like state after I leave this place. My spirit will be like a sleeping princess that will awaken only with the kiss of my Bridegroom who will come to give me eternal life. How long will it be, Father? I do not feel that I can exist without perceiving You. But if I am to have Christian parents, surely they will bring me soon to You. Awaken my spirit as quickly as You will to, Father, for my being longs for You already.

Mother has had ample time to know that my coming is imminent. Her mother and father have arrived and have come together to the hospital from the Ambassador. There is a truce between them—a melancholy peace that remembers the night of Mother's own birth, her measles, her birthdays, her tonsillectomy, her grief when the puppy died, her school plays, her first date with Ben. Each is holding one of Mother's hands now. Each is groping in his mind for a way to pray for her. Aunt Peggy and Uncle Al have prayed aloud with Mother, and she is feeling very peaceful. The social worker from the adoption agency has come too, but after she determined that Mother is not alone emotionally, she has retired to the background.

Mother is praying quietly in her spirit. She knows the Presence of Jesus with her. She has told the social worker that she does want to see me—to count all my fingers and toes, to see if my hair is black like Ben's, to trace the shape of my nose with her finger, to have a picture of my little face in her memory so that when she prays for me every day of her life she will be able to remember me. I must be especially blessed to have *two* mothers who will pray for me.

Frankly, I'm more than a bit reluctant to leave my secure life in this obscure place. I call it obscure because the thick walls of flesh have prevented the people on the outside from seeing the Light that has lived in here with me. All of my needs have been provided with no effort from me. I hope that I will not become so enamored of striving, when I learn how to strive, that I forget my basic and utter dependence on my Father for all of my life and grace.

But He has built abilities and capabilities, capacities and potentials, premises and promises, into my little self. I am eager to get out and stretch, to try myself out, to worship my Creator by imaging Him through my glorious body and mind and spirit. There has never been another image of Him exactly like me. There will never be another. If I do not fulfill His purpose for me, my niche in God's heart will be forever lonely.

With my first lusty breath, the *foramen ovale,* the communication valve between the two sides of my heart, will begin closing permanently. At that time the free communication between Your Spirit and mine will cease, too, and I will be inundated with sensory stimuli that will captivate my attention. Grant,

Father, that my spirit will begin a lifetime quest to reestablish communion with You. Let me be always listening, listening for the quiet voice of Your Spirit. Let me search for You in the Scriptures. Let me see Your glory everywhere in the earth that You have made. Let me be always open and anticipating until that sunburst day when You come to find me.